Get Fit Stay Fit

How to Help Ourselves Live Long and Healthy

Evander Sampson
&
Stephen Small

Stephen's Dedication

I dedicate this book to my wife Dion, who happens to be a nurse, which is very useful when writing a book on the topic of health. Thank you for the many helpful discussions on those key areas of blood circulation, diabetes, and the brain.

Thank you Dion.

TABLE OF CONTENTS

INTRODUCTION

Is this just one more self-help book showing us how to be healthy in body, mind, and spirit? How many more, you might ask!? Well, yes it is, but with additional help on the mental motivation to get fit. We'll leave the spirit to others. The essential point is that it is much easier to find happiness, or if not that, at least a sense of ease, when the body is healthy and exercised. So our focus is on getting physically fit and staying that way for a long and healthy life.

The two authors are Evander Sampson, an experienced and qualified fitness coach who offers guidance in nutrition and exercise, and Stephen Small, who has spent years researching the subject using only scientifically proven advice. A few of the areas under consideration are:

- Weight
- Diet
- Cardio vascular fitness
- Muscular strength
- Brain health
- Motivation
- Exercise and rest
- Gender implications
- Maintaining health in advancing years

We'll be looking at body weight first, as there are health implications to being as thin as a stick or obese. Of course, this brings up the importance of diet and calorie consumption.

The book then leads on to all the other topics listed.

Our whole aim is to help you have a fit body and a motivated mind, and if that helps you have an easier, happier life, then we rejoice in your success!

Testimonies for Evander Sampson

Jennifer is a health professional with type 2 diabetes who was given help by Evander to lose weight on the advice of her doctor. She said,

"Evander, I have been overweight for the last 20 years and have tried many diets but could not get my weight down. I'm overjoyed to have now succeeded in losing 3kg and to have dropped a dress size. Your advice to keep in mind that a slight sense of hunger indicates that I am on a fat-burning cycle has made a huge difference to my motivation. I will keep up with the programme. Thank you so much for your ongoing encouragement."

David, a man approaching retirement, said,

"The most remarkable thing about losing 7kg is that I feel 30 years younger. I can now run up the stairs, and the joy in living just keeps increasing! Thank you, Evander, you have been a great inspiration."

Evander works with individuals to achieve their training goals. These range from weight management and aerobic cardiovascular exercise, to strength training using weights and gym equipment.

He has overcome personal health issues, so he knows from experience the importance of a healthy body.

Together, we share this understanding with anyone who cares to read this book.

WEIGHT

Just one syllable—weight—yet for some, it dominates their waking lives. References to body image are everywhere. Women's magazines have many articles on how to drop a dress size for the summer, and diet fads are ubiquitous. Slim seems to be the in thing—size zero, tall, young, slim women on fashion catwalks can pressurise those concerned about weight.

I, Evander, have just done a quick Google search and come up with so many diets that to list all their names would be tedious, and I do want you to gain something useful from reading this. But just for fun, here are a few— insert the word diet after each. Atkins, Dukan, Kimkins, KE, Mediterranean, South Beach, Stillman, and Weight Watchers are all ways that people choose to eat.

You will come across David in this book, who successfully lost weight. He tells the story of his mother, who was always overweight and always on a diet. It was a rather sad tale in which she rarely succeeded, and if some weight reduction occurred, it was soon put back on. He had come to me because he feared that he was entering a similar cycle. He took my advice, and working together, he did manage to reach his target weight and is maintaining it. So how did he do this? Did he need a special diet? No. The answer was calorie control and following the principles of the Mediterranean diet, which has been scientifically proven to promote health and is recommended by health professionals.

Underweight:

We will come back to the problems of being overweight, but first we will look at the less common problem of being underweight and how that affects health. Being too thin demonstrates why we need food in the first place. So if anyone was wondering, I am not promoting excessive weight reduction. And I can see all too clearly how the media pressures young people—women in particular—to be unhealthily thin.

Anorexia is a real mental problem that in some cases can lead to death. It is often caused by eating too little due to a distorted body image. According to the NHS [1], eating too little will result in problems with muscles and bones. This will include feeling tired and weak. There can be osteoporosis and problems with physical development in children and young adults.

Other parts of the body that are affected include:
- Fertility problems
- Loss of sex drive

In fact, the whole system is affected if there is a lack of calories and essential nutrients. The heart is put under strain by poor circulation, an irregular heartbeat, low blood pressure, heart valve disease, and even heart failure. Neurological problems occur, including brain seizures and memory failure. The whole system can break down with a lack of nutrition, resulting in bowel and kidney failure.

It must be very worrying for a parent to see their teenage daughter lose weight. The fact is that being underweight can kill you—it is as simple as that. At the simplest level, consider the fact that we are warm-blooded mammals who need to maintain a body temperature of 36 degrees Celsius. With the average temperature in the UK being around 10 Celsius, our bodies need to generate heat just to maintain the correct temperature for metabolic processes to continue. This is one of the reasons people prefer to live in houses with central heating, where a comfortable temperature is kept at around 20 °C. It is also why we put on more clothes in cold weather.

Bad things start to happen if our body temperature drops. Hypothermia, a medical emergency requiring hospital treatment, sets in at body temperatures just a few degrees below normal, i.e., below 35 °C [2].

Symptoms of hypothermia are slurred speech, pale, dry skin, and possibly blue lips. Other symptoms are slow breathing, feeling tired, and shivering. People burn calories from food as fuel to keep warm and run this thing called the body. When more calories are "burned" than consumed, the energy must come from somewhere else, which is body fat. When there is insufficient body fat, the body begins to use whatever it can find, beginning with muscle breakdown.

So it is important to have some body fat, but how much? Minimum body fat levels for each individual will depend on gender; for a man, this is 8%, and for a woman, it is 14% [3].

BMI:

This is perhaps the time to introduce a useful yardstick of weight known as the body mass index (BMI). It is just a number calculated using body weight and height that gives an indication of body fat and gives a good correlation.

The formula for the BMI is: weight in kilogrammes divided by height in metres squared. There are many online calculators [4] for the BMI, including those that use weight in stones and pounds and height in feet—very useful for those living in the United States.

BMI ranges

- Low weight – below 18.5
- Healthy – 18.5 to 24.9
- Overweight 25 to 29.9
- Obesity – 30 and over

For my clients, I first assist them in achieving a healthy body weight through calorie control. Once in that range and able to maintain the weight, we work on trying to bring it to a midrange BMI of 22.

As mentioned, the BMI is a yardstick—but a useful one. It gives an individual something to aspire to; they can measure their progress and know when they have achieved their goal. For most people, that is good enough—get in the healthy range and then aim for a BMI of 22. However, if I were training an athlete who was building more muscle mass, knowing that muscle is heavier than fat, a higher BMI would be better. However, for the majority of people, if they can get their BMI into the healthy range—and ideally to 22—then the medical evidence suggests they have a greater chance of staying healthy.

I have discussed the need for food and the importance of avoiding starving ourselves. I will now turn to the more usual problem of people wishing to lose weight.

Overweight:

Let us start with the condition known as obesity—a BMI greater than 30. An individual classified as obese, according to the NHS [5], is at a much higher risk of developing health conditions including:

- Type 2 diabetes
- Hypertension
- Some cancers
- Heart disease
- Stroke
- Liver disease

Not only are there these physical health problems, but there are also mental health issues. Obesity can reduce emotional well being and give rise to poor sleep. Also, obese people can suffer from weight stigma, which consequently reduces their self-esteem.

David—my client, whom we will meet later—feared his weight gain was getting out of hand and that this was making him depressed. The memory of his mother's seemingly constant battle with trying to lose body fat and trying many diets and failing played heavily on David's mind. It was an unhappy childhood experience, and he was determined that in his case he would succeed in not only losing weight but also becoming fitter.

That last point about weight stigma is, I think, rather sad. There is no place in our society for "fat shaming." Unlike some problems such as smoking or alcohol abuse, which we can live without, we have to eat food, and the fact is that eating too much will result in weight gain. As such, controlling calorie intake is certainly problematic for the individual and society as a whole. It is not the case that we can say no to calories—we need them to live.

A TV programme called "My 600-lb. life" about extremely obese individuals trying and often successfully losing weight is very popular. People seem fascinated to the point of obsession with the weight of the human body. It is great when the people on the programme succeed, but I cannot help suspecting the motives of the filmmaker. Is the programme being made to show success in overcoming a difficulty, or is there a large element of prurient voyeurism of other people's distress? I don't know. It is up to each of us to chose how to live. If people are happy being overweight then that is fine. However, if they wish to lose weight, then help can be given.

The TV programme does highlight the difficulties that chronically obese people face. Clothes are made for standard-sized people, so larger sizes may have to be specially made and cost more. Mobility problems occur with all the weight when walking, straining the joints of the back, knees, and ankles. If a heavy person needs to attend the hospital, they may be too large for the equipment. A standard hospital bed is designed to take a person up to approximately 200 kg (440 lb), and therefore obese patients above this figure need a much stronger bed—a bariatric bed. Specialized equipment costs more money, which puts a greater strain on the NHS if it's in the UK. If the overweight patient is in the US or another country, their health insurance is higher, and in some cases, they may not be able to gain health coverage.

Clearly, being obese has its problems. As mentioned, there is no place in a healthy society for fat shaming. Instead, we need to learn about the conditions that leads to weight gain and, in doing so, become empowered to be in control of our food intake.

Our learning starts by considering the role that food plays in daily life. Perhaps one of the greatest pleasures in life is to sit down and eat a good meal with family and friends. Advertisers are aware of this and attempt to entice us to buy their food products—after all, that is their job—and our senses are assaulted. Adverts for food are everywhere—on the TV, on the internet, and on the sides of Sainsbury's, Tesco, and Waitrose trucks. With this ongoing assault on our senses, it is no wonder that the waistline starts to enlarge.

Food can make us feel good, and people who are experiencing low moods can turn to eating to make them feel better. The actor Marlon Brando, once past 30 years old, had a major battle with weight problems. He said that he would visit the refrigerator to find something to make him feel better. Much of his psychological problems stemmed from an unhappy childhood; food simply made him feel better. One young director who had problems getting Marlon on the set would tempt him out of his trailer with food, mainly desserts. Richard Donner said, "Once you fed Marlon, he was in a much better mood" [6].

David, the client, said to me recently that he was annoyed with his own mindless eating. He said, "Yesterday I was stupid; I had sat down late in the evening to watch the news and planned to go straight to bed afterwards—I was not hungry." Next thing I knew, I was eating Pringles, cheese, and a big sandwich. I don't know why; I was not hungry. "I was just being mindless while watching TV."

Then there is the fast food problem. While sitting, pick up the mobile and use an app to get food ("Just Eat" is an example). The only effort is to go to the door to pick up the delivery twenty minutes later. And there it is: a meal full of tasty morsels—and full of calories.

So that gives us a few things to focus our attention on. Let's list them:

- Advertising
- Comfort eating
- Mindless eating
- Ease of obtaining food

We will keep these in mind as we develop a strategy to lose weight. However, the first thing I wish to do is show how to develop the clear motivation necessary to change eating habits and, in so doing, head towards a healthy weight in the normal BMI range and, ideally, a BMI of 22.

We start by first, reviewing the disadvantages of being overweight.

- Health problems

- Feeling unattractive (remember, we're trying to motivate us to lose weight, not to make us feel bad).

- Feeling unhealthy

- Difficulties for society: we wish to avoid setting up problems for the future, which others may have to fix.

- Excessive cost, food itself, clothes, mobility

Secondly, review the advantages of losing weight and being in the normal BMI range. Make a mental note of these.

- Health benefits
- feeling younger and more attractive
- Actually feeling better and having more energy
- Doing our bit for society and hopefully avoiding putting additional strain on others
- Life is less expensive—eating less, wearing standard-size clothes.

Having reviewed the disadvantages of being overweight and motivated ourselves by considering the advantages of a healthy weight, we now turn our attention to healthy eating.

EATING WELL

We have seen that we need food to live, and yet there are so many stories of foods that are harmful—refined sugar, excessive salt, and saturated fats being three of them. We can easily become afraid of eating the calories we need to live. But I do not want to frighten; my aim instead is to help and keep it simple.

Moderation makes sense, and with a few straight-forward principles, we can have a diet that is nutritious, helps towards our fitness goals, and keeps us healthy.

With this in mind, I propose that keeping track of calories and the types of foods we eat be the primary tool for success. The BMI is a good guide. Also, some clients need specific instruction to track calories, but as a starting point, I recommend the NHS Eat Well Guide [7]. This is where the idea of five a day fruit and veg comes in.

Also ensuring the right proportions of protein and carbohydrates are consumed is one of the key elements. This is often illustrated by the get well plate. A simplified version is shown in the pie chart on the next page.

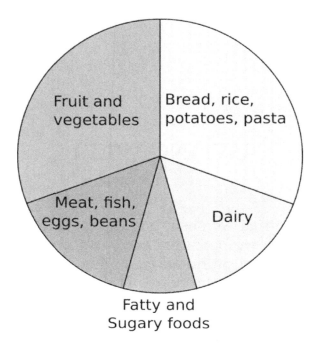

Figure. 1. Eat Well Pie Chart

Calories:

Calories are just a measure of the energy needed to fuel our systems. As we have seen, we are burning calories all the time just to stay warm and keep the body functioning. We can get hungry doing very little, and turn to eating snacks in a mindless manner. This must be avoided. Even if we sit very still, our body is busy doing a job of maintenance and balance, and a basal metabolic rate (BMR) can be calculated depending on gender, age, height, and weight [8]. For a standard man (if there is one), this works out to around 1400 calories per day, while for a woman, it is 1200 calories.

It may be obvious, but I think it needs mentioning: if the calories we use up each day equal what we eat, then our weight stays constant. If we eat more than we need, the extra food becomes fat, and we gain weight. To lose weight, we must consume fewer calories than we burn. Simple!

So how many calories do we need each day?
A general guideline is the following:
For a man, 2500 calories
For a woman, 2000 calories

So, if overweight, try limiting calorie intake to 2000 for men and 1800 for women. This is a good start. Of course, lifestyle and body size (short or tall) play a role. It is worthwhile visiting the online NHS BMI calculator [9], which will give an indication if you are underweight or overweight and make a recommendation of the calorie intake needed to bring the weight into a normal range.

Types of food:

We hear so much about eating five servings of fruit and vegetables a day—why? This is related to the health benefits seen when people eat a Mediterranean-style diet, which includes more fruits and vegetables than a meat-and-carbohydrate-heavy diet. I recommend this diet.

The NHS Why Five a Day online page [10] states the benefits of fruit and vegetables as a good source of vitamins and fiber, which is good for the gut and reduces the incidence of heart disease and cancer.

For a balanced diet, we need carbohydrate, protein, fat, fiber, and minerals.

Carbohydrates are the fuel; they include sugar and starchy foods such as potatoes, pasta, and rice.

Protein is needed to build cells. This nutrient is sourced from animal proteins and vegetables (e.g., soy).

Fat is also a form of energy and helps with cell growth; we need to avoid saturated fats.

Fiber and minerals: fibre helps with digestion, and minerals, including vitamins, are essential for a healthy body; without vitamin C, scurvy develops, and calcium is needed for healthy bones.

So to round this section out, aim for the correct level of calories to control weight. This has its own health benefits. Then ensure that the correct balance of food types is incorporated into the diet. See the 2000-calorie Mediterranean food plan as an example; more meal plans can be found online at Healthline [11].

The meals are designed to offer a balance of protein, healthy fats, and carbohydrates while incorporating a variety of fruits, vegetables, whole grains, and lean sources of protein:

Breakfast (510 calories):

2 scrambled eggs with 1 tsp olive oil (5g) (160 calories)
1 slice whole wheat bread (40g) toasted (110 calories)
1 small avocado (100g) sliced (180 calories)
1 small orange (100g) (60 calories)
1 cup coffee with 1 tbsp low-fat milk (15g) (20 calories)

Lunch (670 calories):

1 can (150g) tuna in water, drained (140 calories)
2 cups mixed greens (100g) (20 calories)
1 medium tomato (150g) sliced (25 calories)
1/2 cucumber (150g) sliced (25 calories)
1/2 cup chickpeas (90g) (80 calories)
1/4 cup crumbled feta cheese (30g) (100 calories)
2 tbsp vinaigrette dressing (30g) (50 calories)
1 whole wheat pita (80g) (220 calories)
1 medium apple (150g) (50 calories)

Dinner (820 calories):

4 oz grilled chicken breast (120g) (125 calories)
1 cup cooked brown rice (195g) (220 calories)
1 cup cooked mixed vegetables (carrots, broccoli, cauliflower) (150g) (75 calories)
2 tbsp hummus (30g) (70 calories)
1/4 cup sliced black olives (30g) (50 calories)
1 tbsp olive oil (15g) (120 calories)
1 medium orange (150g) (60 calories)
1 cup water

Additional Drinks through the day:

2 cups coffee, 3 cups water
1 cup unsweetened almond milk (240ml) (40 calories)
1 cup orange juice (240ml) (110 calories)

Total Calories: 2000

This meal plan provides healthy fats from olive oil, avocado, and almond milk, plenty of fiber and vitamins from fresh fruits and vegetables, lean sources of protein from chicken and tuna, and whole grains like brown rice and whole wheat bread.

Be aware of upcoming social engagements, such as a meal out with friends, and make adjustments to the daily plan.

Vitamins and minerals—do I need a supplement?

The NHS states that we should be able to get all essential vitamins and minerals from our normal diet. Then they go on to say that some people may need supplements [12]. So which is it? Well, it all comes down to the fact that we are all different. For most people eating a varied diet incorporating both animal and vegetable sources, the evidence shows that no supplements are necessary.

A strictly vegan diet can be difficult. The reason is that essential vitamins and nutrients are easier to source from animal products.

Also, there is the interesting case of vitamin D, which we can actually make ourselves when sunlight falls on our skin. There is a problem in the winter months when little sunlight is around. Also, people with darker skin, where their melanocytes successfully ward off the dangers of the sun's rays, find their skin also inhibits the production of vitamin D. This is why African-American and Caribbean people may be recommended a vitamin D supplement.

To know if we are suffering from vitamin deficiency, it is important to get a medical check-up. Some common signs of vitamin deficiency are fatigue, muscle pain, joint aches, brittle nails, etc. But just having these symptoms will not tell us which vitamin is deficient, as they often act throughout the body, affecting many systems. Hence the importance of a medical check-up—getting that blood test done will give the doctor a wealth of information.

Let's have a look at six of the most important vitamins.

Vitamin A
important for vision, healthy skin, and immunity. The body gets it from beta-carotene, the pigment in carrots and other yellowish plants. So it is true that eating carrots improves eyesight.

Vitamin B6
helps to create red blood cells, which are used in the transportation of oxygen. We will see that this oxygen transportation is very important to life itself.

Vitamin B12 (cobalamin)
helps prevent anaemia, improving people's energy levels. Also, it helps keep blood cells healthy, benefits the health of nerve cells, and helps produce DNA.

Vitamin B9 and folic acid
Folic acid reduces neural birth defects like spina bifida and anencephaly. Folic acid also helps our body produce DNA and other genetic material.

Vitamin C
This vitamin is essential for preventing a condition known as scurvy. It helps protect cells, keeping them healthy. Citrus fruits contain vitamin C (ascorbic acid), which is beneficial to our skin, blood vessels, bones, cartilage, and even wound healing. Scurvy was a big problem for the British Navy, as sailors on long sea voyages would become sick. In fact, the use of citrus fruits to help cure scurvy had been considered throughout history, but not enough fresh fruit was carried. What was needed was proof. In 1747, James Lind, a naval surgeon, set up a controlled experiment to find the cause. One group of sailors were given vinegar, another group wine, another cider, and another fresh fruit. The citrus fruit group did not develop scurvy, proving the cause. However, it took a long time for the results of this experiment to be realized, and sailors continued to die as a result. Oh well, that is how things seem to progress: slowly.

Vitamin D
This vitamin interacts with calcium to build strong bones and teeth. It may also aid in the improvement of mood and immunity to disease. Vitamin D deficiency has been associated with some cancers and heart disease.

Vitamin K
This vitamin aids the body's vital role of blood clotting, which may occur as a result of an injury.

Well, that is six vitamins. But there is also mention of minerals; what are they? Minerals are elements from the earth that our bodies need to function well. Many of these minerals are metals, and they are very essential to our health. Here are six necessary minerals that happen to be metals.

Calcium for good bones

Chromium (yes, the shiny metal that is plated onto kettles, toasters, and car bumpers!). This metal helps the body break down fats and carbohydrates.

Iron is needed for red blood cells. I was told as a child that there was enough iron in a body to make a six-inch nail. This was an exaggeration. It is more like a thin, three-inch-long nail weighing one gram.

Magnesium helps with bone health and energy levels.

Potassium helps our body control blood pressure, heart rhythm, hydration, and digestion.

Zinc helps the immune system and is used in wound healing.

So we have all these vitamins and minerals helping us stay healthy and alive. They can all come from a healthy, balanced diet. However, based on my observation of the diet that my clients follow, there may well be a potential for them to miss out and not get enough.

This is particularly difficult when someone is trying to lose weight. They have to balance a reduced calorie intake with the necessity of ensuring nutrient, vitamin, and mineral levels are maintained. It is for this reason—and this is my opinion; others may disagree—that I think it is a good idea for people to consider taking a daily multivitamin tablet.

There is no need to go for an expensive brand like Holland and Barrett. Instead, just go to the local chemist, where there will be a plentiful supply to choose from. Even supermarkets sell multivitamins nowadays. These are often formulated to give a daily dose of all essential vitamins and minerals.

As mentioned, there may be a need for a boost of a particular type—vitamin D comes to mind—to help lift mood in the winter months. Also, for those with darker skin who live in a northern climate, a vitamin D supplement may be necessary all year—there isn't much sun in Britain, I'm afraid. Added to this for myself is a cod liver oil capsule for the valuable Omega 3.

One last note for those on a calorie-controlled diet trying to lose weight: Please do not go into starvation mode. It is very tempting to try to push weight loss at maximum speed.

There is nothing wrong with feeling a little hungry for an hour or so, but if it goes on all day, this is a sure sign that the diet is too extreme. Instead, go for the long haul. Remember, it took a long time to put the weight on, so we can take our time and lose weight gradually. Aim for a half-kilogramme weight loss each week. Ensure enough protein is being consumed, as well as enough fruit and vegetables.

EXERCISE

There are extremes: sedentary, barely moves, desk job, and drives everywhere; favourite position is lying down; and then there's the gym-goer who trains five hours a day, has rippling muscles, and good vascular fitness, but requires 3000 calories per day to maintain this fitness.

Exercise is not needed to lose weight, but it can help as it will burn calories. Consider this: as mentioned, the BMR for a man is 1400 calories a day if he does absolutely no exercise. So if this man limits his diet to 1300 calories a day and does no exercise whatsoever, he will slowly lose weight.

David did not want to do exercise to start with and at first relied simply on reduced calorie intake to lose weight—and it worked! He did later work on exercise and started by simply going for a walk, progressing to riding his bike, and only now is he working on some aerobic exercise to improve his cardio-vascular fitness.

Couch sitting and weight training are examples of lower and upper levels of exercise. Most of us wish to be somewhere in the middle of these extremes. So our first mission is to think carefully and see what level of weight and physical fitness we want. Perhaps we are a little overweight. We may like the idea of going to the gym every day, but our lives do not allow it.

For example, a young couple raising their newborn child will be devoting a large portion of their lives to this role, so what they need or want is to incorporate an exercise routine into their day-to-day lives. They may feel that a static bike in the home works well for exercise and that they can motivate each other by sharing responsibilities and allowing time for the other to exercise.

CASE STUDY: DAVID

Because all our lives are different, when I meet someone for the first time, I always ask them about their lifestyle and what they want to achieve. Our first case study illustrates this. David came to me and said he wanted to get fit and lose weight. Well, I knew the direction he wanted to go, but that was all I knew; more detail was needed. So I asked him about his health and why he wanted to lose weight, and after some discussion, he came up with the following:

Age: 64 and about to retire

High cholesterol and a BMI of slightly more than 27.

Exercise level: low; he has sedentary interests (as a computer whiz), where sitting down and clicking a mouse does not use many calories. He does have a garage where he makes wooden items with hand tools. He drives everywhere instead of walking.

He believes his diet is adequate, but he wants to increase the amount of fruits and vegetables while decreasing the amount of carbohydrates. He drinks around four bottles of beer each week.

He said he wanted to be fit for health reasons, particularly the heart, and within the normal BMI range of 18.5 to 24.9.

We came up with the following:
Reduce weight, aim for a BMI of 24, and in so doing improve cardiovascular fitness.
For his height, this means reducing his weight from 76 kg to 70 kg.

To achieve this, we used SMART goals.

- S - Specific: losing weight to a predetermined level in a given amount of time.

- M - Measurable: weight loss of 7 kg

- A - Achievable: Weight loss is possible but not excessive.

- R - Relevant: It makes sense to lose this weight and is appropriate for this person.

- T - Time-based: We decided to achieve the goal by his 66th birthday, which is on April 23, 2023, after starting the programme in January 2022. So aim to get to 70 kg by this date, but ideally earlier so as to have some time to stabilise the weight. This weight loss is less than 0.5 kg per month.

Following NHS guidelines, we came up with the following combination of diet and exercise:

Diet: Begin with a daily 2000-calorie diet rich in fibre from fruits and vegetables; follow the Eat Well Guide. Reduce alcohol consumption to two small bottled beers each week.

Exercise: He did not want to visit a gym or go swimming. So we decided that walking more than driving would be the best option. When he was out walking, he would try to do it briskly so that his heart rate would rise. As David is also a keen woodworker and has his own carpentry shop, this was an opportunity for exercise. Rather than use power tools, David said he would instead saw, plane, and chisel by hand.

The need to plan and keep a record:

For this to succeed, two documents are needed.

- The diet plan was laid out one week in advance: breakfast, break time, lunch, and dinner.

- A weekly record of weight. This can be on paper or in a spreadsheet and include a graph of weight gain or loss each week. I suggested he weigh himself once a week, for example, after waking up on Sunday morning, and record the weight on the graph.

David decided to keep a spreadsheet. He bought himself an electronic weighing scale that also gave a calculation of his BMI, water percentage, fat percentage, and bone density. David thought that having all this information presented to him each Sunday morning would be an incentive for the following week. The model of weighing scale he bought was found on Amazon.uk. Just search "BMI weighing machine" to find many similar models.

I advised David to keep a notebook of his exercise and diet—the things that worked well and the occasions when difficulties occurred.

My other piece of advice was to make adjustments as needed—if a kilogramme has not been lost after one month, reduce calorie intake to 1800 per day and/or increase the amount of exercise.

We had ongoing conversations at key points in 2022, particularly when David was having difficulties. He produced the chart below showing the weight loss up until February 2023.

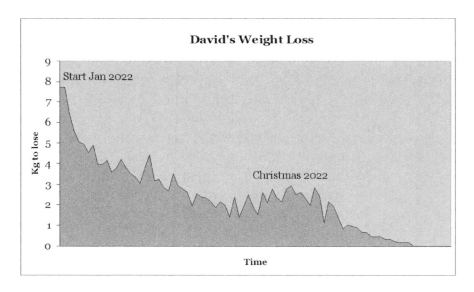

Figure. 2

Here is an interview with David in February 2023: 13 months after starting the diet (2 months left on the plan).

E is myself, Evander
D is David.

E: Hello, David.
D: Hello Evander,

E: Can you tell me about your experience so far? What is your current weight?

D: I have been encouraged by the advice to take my time to lose the weight. I've now lost about 7 kg, or a stone in British terms. The most amazing thing that I did not expect is that I actually feel so much lighter and younger. Instead of 65, I feel like I am in my thirties. It is so much easier to climb a flight of stairs because I do not have to carry an extra 7 kg of fat with me. I now weigh 70.5 kg, or 11 st 1 lb. I am so near but seem to be bouncing up and down with the weight.

E: That's fantastic news, David. You are so close to your target weight of 70 kg, or 11 st, and you have done this in just over a year. You have another two months to achieve that last half Kg and then hold the weight. Do you know what is making this last bit difficult?

D: Thank you for your encouragement, Evander, it is most appreciated. I do feel I have done well with the diet, but less so with the exercise. I am still sedentary. I do take walks, but not every day. So I am dependent on calorie reduction in my diet to lower my weight. My danger zones, or rather, times, are well known to me. Looking at my spreadsheet, I can see where the weight went up. It is nearly always on a special occasion such as Christmas, my birthday, or being invited to stay at a friend's house for a few days. When these events occur, I tend to eat more and am encouraged to do so by others. However, afterwards, I feel despondent, as I know I have overeaten and have set myself back a week. This despondency shows itself after the event because I find it takes me a few days to re-establish my diet routine. It is as if I have become a bit fed up (no pun intended) with it all.

E: That is interesting that these life events break up your routine. You say you find it discouraging when the weight goes up. Have you found a solution to this?

D: As I said, I did at first get despondent when the weight went up. It was annoying to have worked hard to maintain the diet and find I had lost a kilogram, only to put it back on when invited out. There is a social pressure to eat the food provided, and I do not like to offend. But there has been a difference in my thinking of late. I now see it just as a process. If I accept these invitations, then I am likely to gain weight. This last Christmas and the cold weather was difficult and I ate too much. This can be seen on the chart. What I am aiming to do in the future is be clear with people that I want to maintain my diet when I am with them and ask that they be understanding. I do not want to be overly strict or antisocial, but I can say no to the pudding and the glass of wine at the end of the meal.

E: It sounds like you have a plan, and I wish you all the best going forward. How have you found the discipline of weighing once a week?

D: Getting on the scales every Sunday morning is just great—and that is the only time I weigh. I really look forward to seeing the weight and am getting pretty good at knowing if I have gained or lost before I step on the machine. The weighing scales that provide BMI, fat, water, and bone density also keep my attention. So if I lose weight one week, I can see immediately the change in the BMI, which is also encouraging for the reduction in fat percentage. I also enjoy entering the information each week into the spreadsheet and seeing the effect on the graph, hopefully going downward. This fits very well with my interest in computers. One other thing I do to aid motivation is watch YouTube videos of people who have achieved their weight loss goals. These are really uplifting to watch.

E: So you have two months left of this weight loss plan. "What are you going to prioritize: exercise or diet?"

D: I am definitely going to concentrate on the diet and feel very confident that I will reach my target weight and hold it there. In fact, my aim is to achieve this in the next month and then spend the rest of the time stabilising and improving the diet. In particular, I wish to reduce the alcohol consumption further—go from two or three bottles of beer a week to just one at the weekend. I also want to eat more vegetarian food without being overly strict about it. I am also aiming to reduce my milk consumption, as this is a surprising source of calories. I may drink black coffee.

E: But what about exercise?

D: I find exercise difficult to incorporate into my life, but I do realise the importance of this for my health. I know I can reach my goal weight through diet alone. In fact, it has reached the point now that I do not need to make meal plans. I know roughly how many calories I consume each day and try to keep it under 1500. When we come to April and I have reached my goal weight and am confident that I can hold it there, can we then decide on the next health direction? I just feel like I want to get the weight down at the moment.

E: Yes, of course we can. Let's see where you are in April and set another goal at that point. I am very inspired by your confidence and wish you every success. I think we will stop the interview there. If you want to talk about anything, please contact me by phone, text, Facebook, or whatever method you prefer.

D: Thank you very much, Evander. You have been a great inspiration. I will certainly call for advice if needed.

MOTIVATION

Motivation is required to stay fit and maintain a healthy body weight. As David mentioned, when his weight rose, he at first became despondent. This reduced motivation unsettled his routine, and it took him a few days to re-establish his diet.

It is very important to stay motivated. While working towards the goal, that picture of our new body needs to burn bright in the mind. Using David's experience, he mentioned that he is motivated by watching YouTube videos of others who have succeeded at getting to their target weight. This may not work for everyone, so we need to observe our own mind and behaviour. We need to find out what works for us.

For myself, I like to reflect on the benefits of being at the correct weight and feeling physically fit.
I emphasise the following benefits for myself:

Increased energy levels

The importance to my health. I had problems with my lungs as a child and this area of my system is weak. By being fit and at the right weight, I am not putting too great a strain on my lungs.

Greater alertness

Just feeling good—greater self-esteem

The buzz that comes from exercise—the release of endorphins—is why I exercise at the gym five days a week. Exercise reduces the risk of heart and vascular disease.

To motivate myself, I like to go over these benefits in my mind and repeat them like a mantra.

Like David, I enjoy watching motivational videos on exercise and diet, which are abundant on YouTube. Or just go for straight motivation. One I like is by Arnold Schwarzenegger [13], where he points out not to be afraid to fail.

David did not always lose his 1 kg per month, but there was no need to be disheartened. Instead, it was a case of taking stock and seeing what to change. He saw for himself the dangers of accepting too many social engagements where family and friends would encourage him to eat more calories than his diet allowed. He is working on being clear with people that he wishes to keep to his calorie limit. This is a great understanding of how to stay motivated.

I would like to see David walk and exercise more often, as I know this will benefit his health. But I am also mindful of the fact that he must be willing to do this, and at the moment he has stated that he can reach his goal with diet alone. I must respect his wish. My guess is that once he reaches his target weight and feels confident that he can hold it, he will then want to set other health goals.

This has been my experience. If I give someone too much to do in one sitting, they may become disheartened and fail to meet their goals. It is much better to achieve one goal, then take stock and set another. By doing this, people are able to achieve things that they once thought impossible.

Assuming David achieves his weight loss goal, I can guarantee that he will be motivated by this success. "What next?" will then be the question. He may be motivated to stay just where he is with weight and exercise, and that will be just fine. However, I do believe he can achieve more. At this point, I will suggest (only suggest) that he consider setting more goals.

These goals are:

- Aim to increase the weight loss and stop at a mid-BMI of 22, which for David's height is a weight of 64 kg or about 10 stone. So there's another 6 kg to go. I will, however, emphasise to David that he is already within a healthy BMI range and that any weight between 64 and 70 kg is perfectly fine for him. Success will be measured by staying within this range. And if he just reaches the BMI of 22, even once this gets an A, the A+ will be maintenance of this mid-range BMI.

- Increase cardio-vascular fitness. This can be achieved by brisk walking, riding his bicycle, and swimming. I will try to "sell" this exercise increase to David by pointing out that he will have a greater sense of physical ease, coupled with more energy and alertness. I will state how this cardio-vascular fitness can be measured and how it can be incorporated into his spreadsheet, thereby using his interest in computing to motivate him.

- Diet: David expressed a wish to move to a more vegetarian diet and also reduce alcohol consumption to one beer each week. I will suggest that we look into the health benefits of this and learn about the pros and cons before embarking. Remember that all of this highlighting of benefits is intended to increase motivation. He may wish to keep to some animal products, such as fish, eggs, and chicken, for essential protein. The goal here will be to have two weeks of each month alcohol-free and to avoid red meat such as beef when in his house—i.e., success is zero beef in a three-month period.

- Every Sunday, he weighs himself. Cardiovascular measurements are to be decided. Consideration will be given to the technology that enables the recording of his pulse, blood pressure, breathing rate, and number of daily steps. This also should help motivate David, as it will leverage his interest in such technology.

Well, all this is in the future. David has to achieve his first goal by April 2023 and then see if he wishes to go further as described above. As mentioned, it is David's choice, and if he wishes to just stay at his first goal of reaching 70 kg, that is just fine. We will see how it goes.

With this section being all about motivation, we can consider all the things that help. I have been talking about exercise above, but what about rest and relaxation? There are other considerations for health such as personal hygiene, and the science behind sleep in particular is remarkable.

SLEEP

Any change we make to our lifestyle is a challenge, and we need energy, organization, and drive to achieve it. A good habitual pattern of sleep helps us greatly in our endeavour.

Recent scientific studies are showing just how beneficial sleep is to our wellbeing. Sleep is essential for health. During sleep, our body makes repairs that keep us healthy, and so the quantity and quality of sleep have a great effect on our mental and physical wellbeing.

People can feel cranky if they have not slept well. Studies have shown that a chronic lack of sleep can lead to anxiety, depression, and irritability. So it makes sense to put some time and effort into establishing a good sleep routine.

We are back to the motivation side of things again. Consider how good sleep improves cardiac health. During sleep, our heart rate slows, with a consequent reduction in blood pressure, giving the whole circulation system a bit of a rest.

Sleep also affects the body's ability to use insulin, the regulator of glucose absorption. This is very important for all of us, but in particular for those with a diabetic condition. Having a good night's sleep helps with blood sugar regulation. Consequently, it has been found that people who have reduced sleep on a consistent basis are at a higher risk of developing type 2 diabetes.

The physical effects of good sleep on brain function are becoming more clear. With enough sleep, we can think clearly, remember well, learn effectively, and maintain good brain function throughout our waking hours. Studies have shown that people who have had poor sleep perform poorly during multi-tasking activities.

There are also benefits to good sleep as we get older. Sleep repairs the body and produces growth hormones. These growth hormones aid in the repair of tissues and cells throughout life, even in old age. Sleep improves the body's reaction to infection.

We can see that it is important to get good sleep. So sleep is another element that needs careful management. It is as important as healthy eating and getting the right amount of exercise. Sleep also helps us maintain a healthy weight as it promotes leptin, the appetite-suppressing hormone. Consequently, with poor sleep, there can be a greater sense of hunger and the potential to eat more than needed.

Developing good habits is the key to getting a good night's sleep. Try to get 8 hours of sleep each night, and because it takes some time to relax into sleep, I recommend 9 hours. Keeping regular hours establishes the habit of getting enough sleep, and it becomes easier.

If you're feeling tired during the day, feel free to take a 20-minute power nap. The bedroom should be cool, dark, and, above all, quiet. The bed should be comfortable. The old idea of a hard mattress being good for us has been discredited as it can give rise to back pain. Avoid stimulants before going to bed, particularly coffee or tea, which contain caffeine.

Try to avoid over stimulating mental activity just before sleep. A light read may be OK, but try to put the phone and laptop to one side and switch them off. More sleep tips can be found at the sleep foundation website [14].

Concluding this section, I suggest keeping the benefits of good sleep and the disadvantages of poor sleep close to our minds—again, this will help with motivation. Look at the NHS link [15]. Keep it simple. Good sleep patterns promote a sense of wellbeing and increased mental clarity. Conversely, poor sleep leads to low mood, confusion, and being at increased risk of obesity, diabetes, and heart diseases, which all shorten life expectancy.

HYGIENE

David told me of his time as a little boy. He was always a bit grubby and did not like to wash very much, yet he was rarely ill. However, the boy up the road, who was never allowed out, always seemed to be having colds, yet he was so clean! David just could not understand it. Well, the main covering of our body is the skin, and it does a very good job of protecting us from infection. So this may have protected David. Of course, now that he is a grown man, he has a shower once a day and looks like a very neat and tidy older man.

Oral hygiene may be more problematic for health. David has been telling me that since the COVID outbreak he has not been able to see a dentist and that his teeth hurt. I mentioned to him that there may well be a link between oral health and heart disease. He said he had never heard of this before, which prompted me to question my own understanding and review the evidence.

Stephen my co author came up with some useful data. According to the mayoclinic [16] there may be some connection between oral health and heart disease, although this has not been proven.

Studies have shown:

- Gum disease is linked to an increased risk of developing heart disease.
- Poor dental health increases the risk of a bacterial infection in the blood stream, which can affect the heart valves.
- Tooth loss has been linked to cardiovascular disease.
- A connection exists between diabetes and cardiovascular disease. Also, people with diabetes benefit from good oral health treatment.

Recommendations for oral health

- At least twice a day, brush your teeth.
- Floss daily.
- Schedule regular dental checkups and cleanings.

ALCOHOL CONSUMPTION

I am not suggesting a necessity for abstinence. Alcohol in moderation provides a way for some people to wind down, and a glass of wine over a meal with friends is one of the delights of life. Studies have shown that red wine can reduce blood pressure. But alcoholic drinks contain calories; according to the NHS, "drinking 5 pints of lager a week adds up to 44,200 kcal over a year, equivalent to eating 221 doughnuts."

Another thing to consider with alcohol is that with consumption, our resolve can weaken, and when we are trying to get fit or alter our weight, we need all the resolve and drive we can muster.

So, my recommendation is to stick to the NHS guidelines of 14 units per week and try to limit your alcohol consumption.

For reference, 14 units are equivalent to 6 pints of average-strength beer or 10 small glasses of low-strength wine.

If we return to David for a moment, he has successfully reduced his alcohol consumption from four bottles of beer a week to two, which is a reduction of approximately 500 calories for the week. He does not want to give up alcohol entirely, but he does want to limit himself to one bottle on weekends. If he succeeds with this, it will be a reduction of 750 calories a week. This is significant as it amounts to about half a day's food allowance per week and can only help his weight loss goals.

CARDIO VASCULAR FITNESS

Our focus so far has been on weight control using diet, pointing to the benefits of sleep, and reducing alcohol consumption. I now turn to physical fitness, and in particular cardiovascular fitness, for this will enable us to live and stay healthy.

Let's start by defining our terms. Cardio—a word from the Greek, Kardia—literally means the heart. Vascular is from Latin, "Vasculum," a small vessel, and from Modern Latin, "Vascularis," relating to tubes. The heart is simply a pump that pushes blood around the body through the vascular system.

As I sit here, I am placing my right forefinger on my left wrist and can feel a pulse as the artery (which carries blood from the heart) expands and contracts in line with the beat of the heart. It expands and can be felt because the pressure changes with each beat.

As the heart pumps, the pressure in the artery system increases, and while the heart is getting ready for the next beat, it decreases. Both of these pressures can be measured as systolic (the high beating one) and diastolic (the lower resting one). Because the artery is somewhat elastic and expands and contracts with changing pressure, I can feel the heartbeat (the pulse) in my wrist. The pulse rate in my case at the moment is 62 beats per minute, which is fairly good for a resting phase—after all, I am just typing.

So the heart creates the blood pressure, which is needed in the body to move the fluid—blood—around our system.

Normal blood pressure for most adults will be less than 120 systolic and less than 80 diastolic if we have a good, efficient cardio- and vascular system. The numbers refer to millimetres of mercury—literally the pressure needed to raise a column of mercury a vertical distance. In older movies, when a doctor took the blood pressure, he would have an inflatable cuff, which he would pump up and listen to with a stethoscope at the elbow for the sounds of blood flow. The doctor would observe the mercury column while listening to determine the systolic and diastolic pressures.

It is much simpler nowadays as we can just use an electronic device at home; however, the need for an inflatable cuff has continued.

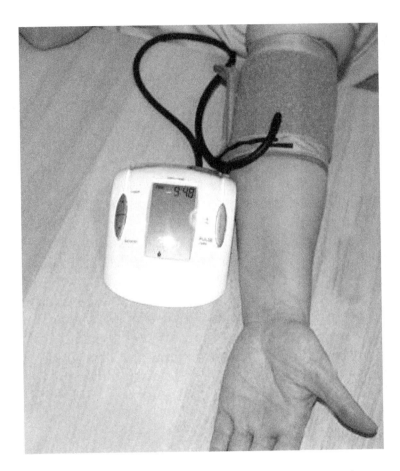

Figure. 3. Electronic blood pressure monitor

I want to go into some detail here about the cardiovascular system and why it is so important. We will see that it is not just the heart and vascular system that are involved but also the lungs.

For now, just hold the picture of an efficient pump—the heart pushing blood around the body through the vascular system. I should also add that the vascular system also involves the lymphatic system. The lymph tubes carry lymphatic fluid (containing water and blood cells). This system helps protect and maintain the fluid quality of the body by filtering and draining lymph from bodily regions.

We will concentrate on the fluid called blood. What is it needed for? Clearly, if it is valuable stuff and is needed in different parts of the body, then it is important to have a good transport system, which is where the cardio-vascular bit comes in. If the heart is weak or the tubes are clogged or not very flexible, then we can expect problems.

Blood is the transport fluid that carries oxygen and nutrients to the body organs that need them. Blood does other important things. Waste materials from the body tissues are filtered out in the kidneys and leave the body in the form of urine. Also, the body's temperature is controlled by the flow of blood among the different parts of the body. This is needed because heat is generated by the body as it breaks down nutrients for energy, makes new tissue, and gives up waste matter.

On arrival at an organ such as a muscle, it is the cells of that muscle that offload the nutrients and oxygen and put back into the blood the waste products for elimination. As an analogy, think of a delivery driver from a supermarket using the efficient road network to bring much-needed food to a home that houses growing children. This road network isn't just for transporting goods. The refuse driver uses the same network to come and pick up the trash discarded by this family. If the roads are being dug up, if the driver goes sick, or if his van breaks down, then this family will go hungry, and waste products will build up. We don't want anyone to go hungry! Similarly, in the cardiovascular system, we don't want any organ to be starved of oxygen and nutrients.

The nutrient side of the CV system is easy enough to follow as blood picks up nutrients from the digestive system. Once in the blood, and as the blood is moving, nutrients are transported to where they are needed.

However, where does oxygen come in? All functions of the body, such as digesting food, moving muscles, and thinking, need oxygen. Gas exchange occurs throughout the body as red blood cells in the blood give up oxygen while carbon dioxide reattaches to these cells as a waste product. Our lungs are responsible for providing oxygen to our bodies and eliminating waste gases like carbon dioxide. Oxygen is so important that in the book "How We Die" by Sherwin B. Nuland [17], he states that all death is due to a lack of oxygen in one form or another.

So how does oxygen get from the lungs to the blood? It is the heart that does this. I mentioned how the heart is a pump. However, it turns out that there are two pumps.
The right side of the heart pumps blood to the lungs, where it picks up oxygen before returning to the left side of the heart. From here, oxygenated blood is pumped out to the rest of the body. It moves through the large arteries, then smaller ones. Then the blood finds its way to the small capillary vessels, where it departs with its nutrients and oxygen for the various organs.

The blood picks up the waste products, including the carbon dioxide, and finds itself draining from the capillaries into the veins and returning to the right side of the heart. This blood is then pumped again to the lungs for elimination of the carbon dioxide and replenishment with life-giving oxygen. The heart keeps doing this for as long as we live.

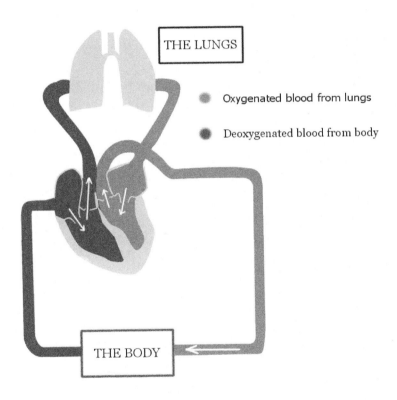

THE LUNGS

Oxygenated blood from lungs

Deoxygenated blood from body

THE BODY

Figure. 4. The Heart Circulation

As most of us want to live long, healthy lives, it makes sense to keep this CV system in tip-top condition. Unfortunately, there are many things that can go wrong and result in us becoming unfit for work. Think of vascular disease affecting efficient blood flow either by blocking or weakening blood vessels or by damaging the valves that are found in veins. And because our body organs need nutrients and oxygen, it is clear how body structures are damaged by vascular disease. If the blood cannot flow the organs are not adequately supplied, and the system can break down.

So just think: how do we keep the blood flowing and efficiently depositing oxygen and nutrients while collecting and eliminating waste products? As we have seen, it is a complex system involving the heart, the tubes (arteries and veins), and the lungs. All of these parts need to be healthy. Using the analogy of the delivery driver, if the engine of the vehicle breaks down, the roads are impassable, or the petrol station is starved of fuel, those little children will not get any food, and the trash will pile up.

How to keep the CV system healthy

We will divide it up into its component parts.

Heart

This double pump is a muscular bag with two inlets and two outlets. When the muscular pump operates, blood flows in one direction only—to the lungs on the right side and the rest of the body on the left side. It is the valves in the heart that control the direction of flow. As the blood flows out of the left side, through the aorta, it first branches into small arteries that feed the heart muscle itself—known as the coronary arteries.

Coronary comes from the Latin coronaries, meaning "crown," which is an apt name as these are very important vessels like a crown over the heart—they must be kept clear to allow the blood to flow. A heart attack (coronary) is when a blockage occurs in a coronary artery and the heart muscle it feeds is starved of oxygen and nutrients. The muscle, then so starved, can no longer function, and the pump—the heart—fails. The narrowing of arteries is known as atherosclerosis.

Many factors can cause these coronary arteries to narrow and block; more information can be found online via this NHS link [18].

In summary, coronary heart disease (CHD) is most often due to a build-up of fatty deposits (atheroma) on the inside walls of the coronary arteries. This atherosclerosis can have many causes, as listed.

- Smoking
- High blood pressure
- High cholesterol
- Lack of exercise
- Diabetes
- Being obese

Taking a look at each of these risk factors,

Smoking brings nicotine and carbon monoxide into the blood stream, which causes a strain on the heart by making it work faster—for example, we want carbon monoxide out of the body, not in, so the heart needs to work more to get rid of this. Also, other chemicals damage the lining of our coronary arteries, all of which can lead to blood clots.

High blood pressure (hypertension) puts a strain on our heart and vascular system—the tubes become less elastic and narrower, and it takes much more effort for the heart to pump blood.

Cholesterol is a fat that is needed for body cells, but an excess amount can increase the risk of deposits in the arteries and hence a narrowing and lower vascular efficiency.

Lack of exercise increases the likelihood that deposits build up in the arteries, again making them narrow.

Inactivity allows fatty deposits to build up in arteries. To keep those arteries clear and healthy, exercise helps greatly. I will talk about exercise later, but good information is provided by the NHS [19].

Diabetes can lead to CHD as it promotes the lining of blood vessels to become thicker, restricting blood flow.

Obesity, just being overweight puts a greater strain on the heart. At the simplest level, the body as a machine is less efficient as a larger body than needed is being maintained and carried about.

So there we are—there are many bad habits and conditions that can narrow the coronary arteries around the heart, with the corresponding result that the heart has to work harder. Before I look in detail at health advice such as an exercise routine, we will look at the other components of the cardiovascular system. Next, we look at the lungs: how they work, how they can be damaged, and how to keep them healthy.

Lungs

As mentioned, lungs enable oxygen to enter the bloodstream and carbon dioxide to exit the body. My own lungs were very weak when I was young and I have had to work to keep my body healthy. As we breathe in, air flows down our windpipe and enters our left and right lungs. Further branching takes place until the final destination of the air sacs (alveoli) is reached. Alveoli are like thin-walled balloons, but very small. In the walls of these alveoli, blood is flowing through small capillaries. The walls are so thin that oxygen can pass through them and enter the red blood cells, while carbon dioxide passes out and into the alveoli. On exhalation, this waste carbon dioxide is expelled from the body. Now the oxygen-enriched blood returns to the left side of the heart, where it is pumped to the rest of the body.

Weakening of the cardiovascular system at the lungs occurs when this gaseous exchange is impaired. So if the alveoli are coated with pollution or tars and chemicals from cigarette smoke, gas exchange is less efficient.

A good analogy is that of an air filter, such as in a tumble dryer. Fibres from clothing push up against the filter and reduce the efficiency of the air getting through. The consequence is that the clothes take longer to dry. This is why we periodically clean the filter by removing the fluff that has built up. But here the analogy with the lungs breaks down, for we cannot easily get into our body and clean the lungs.

Fortunately, there are some things we can do to promote lung health.

Stop smoking, or even better, don't start!

Cigarette smoking is the major cause of lung cancer and chronic obstructive pulmonary disease (COPD), which includes chronic bronchitis and emphysema. Not only does it coat the alveoli with chemicals, it also causes inflammation, which promotes bronchitis. Cigarette smoke damages lung tissue, causing cellular changes that develop into cancer. Try also to avoid areas of air pollution; the countryside is better than a busy road.

Drink plenty of water (tea, coffee, and diluted juices are also fine); about 6 to 8 cups should be spread throughout the day. This helps the lungs, as they need hydration to keep the mucous lining from getting too thick and reducing gas exchange. We are constantly losing body water, which makes up about two-thirds of our body weight. The lungs help regulate our hydration level. Not only do we breathe out carbon dioxide, we also breathe out moist air. Our kidneys excrete water with urine, and our skin loses hydration via sweat. A clear sign of lack of hydration is a dry mouth, coupled with a sense of thirst and darker than normal urine. We must spread our fluid intake throughout the day, as drinking too much water in one sitting can cause problems such as decreased sodium levels in brain cells.

Eat a healthy diet high in fruits and vegetables. These have antioxidant properties that help the cellular structure of the lungs. Also, eating high-protein foods helps lung function. Lean chicken or other meats, eggs, milk, and fish will all be helpful. Soya is a good source of vegetable protein for those moving towards a vegetarian style of diet.

Also, damage to the muscular systems that aid breathing—e.g., the diaphragm and the intercostal muscles between the ribs—can hamper gaseous exchange. Imagine a bruised rib where breathing becomes painful— the person breathes in a shallow manner, and their blood oxygen level decreases. Therefore, strengthening the muscular system that aids breathing is valuable and was one of the main things that improved my blood oxygen level. This can be done in a number of ways.

Just keep active. A brisk walk, swimming, or low-weight lifting can all help. The idea is to get the pulse rate up along with the breathing rate. As the main muscle involved in breathing is the diaphragm, it makes sense to strengthen and develop its efficiency. The diaphragm is a dome-shaped area of muscle across the bottom of our ribcage. It is the main muscle involved in our breathing. When we inhale, this is because the diaphragm is contracting. This forces the lungs to expand, creating a negative pressure that pulls air in through the nose and mouth. When we exhale, the diaphragm relaxes and moves upward, which pushes air out of the lungs and out through our mouth and nose.

The diaphragm normally moves automatically, but it is of course possible to bring it under conscious control. For example, I am holding my breath right now until the urge to take another breath is just too strong. We can strengthen the diaphragm by doing belly breathing. This is a deep breathing technique that can make the diaphragm contract and relax more than normal. It makes us breathe very deeply, bringing in a full lung of air and then puffing it all out, getting rid of the stale air lurking at the bottom.

A deep breathing exercise is a very good way to start the day. Sit down and bring attention to the rise and fall of the abdomen—a sensation felt just above the navel. Now take a deep breath all the way in while pushing the belly out. Hold that for a few seconds, then breathe out and pull the belly up so that the lungs are emptied. Hold that empty state for a second or two, and then repeat the cycle. Aim to do this for around 20 breaths. You will then have a healthy amount of oxygen in your bloodstream with which to go on with your day.

Laugh more. Laughter has many health benefits. It is similar to deep belly breathing—think belly laugh. By taking deeper breaths and longer exhalations, this keeps our lungs healthy and flushes stale air from them. Laughing rids the lungs of residual air.

Sit upright. Good posture, where we sit or stand upright, enables improved respiratory function. This overcomes the dangers of long sitting as it strengthens and stabilises the core as we maintain a good fight against the forces of gravity.

Sing at the local church or with friends and family. This is a bit like deep belly breathing and laughing—just getting more air in and out of the body. Also, it makes us feel good, and there is nothing wrong with that.

Having looked at the heart and lungs, we now move on to the third component of CVD—the vascular system.

Vascular System

Let us assume we have a healthy heart pumping a sufficient quantity of blood. Also, the lungs are performing well by passing oxygen into the blood and taking carbon dioxide out. What we now need is a set of tubes to take this oxygenated blood around the body. This is where the vascular system comes in.

Basically, the carrying of oxygenated blood to the body starts at the largest and strongest artery—the aorta— which is the largest diameter and strongest of all the blood-carrying tubes. It then branches and flows into smaller arteries until it reaches the fine capillary tubes in the organs of the body. Exchanges of oxygen, carbon dioxide, nutrients, and waste take place. Then the deoxygenated blood, at much lower pressure, drains into larger vessels called veins. These have a small diameter at the start and grow larger as they find their way back to the heart. Consider a river system: small springs, streams, and brooks feed into rivers, which then feed into larger rivers, until a large mass of water flows to the sea.

Things can go wrong with arteries, capillaries, and veins— all of which affect CVD. We will look at each component individually and how to keep them healthy. This is a vast subject, and I am only pointing out the essentials here. Fortunately, the recommendations for health are similar to those for the heart and lungs. Having said that, I think it is good to have an overview of how the system works— and, moreover, how it can fail.

Arteries

The arteries need to be strong as they carry the higher pressures while also being elastic. As mentioned before, a build up of plaque that narrows the interior diameter of the artery will reduce blood flow and put a greater strain on the heart. Also, this material can break away and block an artery, cutting off the needed blood supply to an organ. This can result in amputation. It is also responsible for heart attacks and strokes. Health is all about keeping the blood flowing.

Capillaries

These very small diameter blood vessels—5 to 10 micrometres—are the working end of the system. Their walls are so thin that molecules of oxygen, carbon dioxide, water, and many others can pass through them via osmosis. As long as blood can get to them, they function well. Diabetes is a particular issue because high blood sugar levels reduce the elasticity of all blood vessels. This can make them narrow and reduce blood flow. And as we have seen, this narrowing increases the risk of high blood pressure and damage to large and small blood vessels. As the capillaries are small, there is a particular problem for the eyes because impairment of blood flow to the retinal area can cause blindness. Also, the extremities, such as the toes, are particularly prone to diabetic damage, as a lack of blood flow here can lead to a requirement for amputation.

Veins

Veins are flexible, hollow tubes with valves, allowing flow in only one direction. Valves are needed as there is little blood pressure in the veins. If a vein is cut, the blood just oozes out, while an artery pumps it out. When our muscles contract, the veins are squashed, the one-way valves open, and blood moves through our veins. When our muscles relax, the valves close, which prevents the blood from flowing backwards.

If the valves inside our veins become damaged, they may leak and allow blood to flow backwards. This can cause a pool of blood to form, causing the veins to swell. The bulging veins are called varicose; they can be seen as lumps under the skin. The problem for health is that the blood moves slowly and sticks to the inside of the veins. The swelling may be noticed first, along with itching, a throbbing sensation, and the potential for blood clots.

As always, the major problem is that the flow of blood from the veins is restricted, particularly from the legs to the heart. We need to keep the blood flowing.

Fortunately, the way to prevent CVD is the same for the heart, lungs, and vascular system. And, because repetition helps us remember things, here are some ways to stay healthy.

Avoid smoking and pollution; this will increase lung efficiency.

Keep blood pressure in the healthy range of 80–120 mm Hg to prevent arterial strain and keep them open.

Keep cholesterol at a healthy level so that it does not build up in the vascular system.

Increase the heart rate and breathing rate through exercise. A brisk walk and swimming are recommended, but more details are to follow.

Eat well with a good balance of carbohydrates, protein, fat, fibre, vitamins, and minerals. The Mediterranean diet is recommended; again, details are to follow.

- Stay hydrated
- Breathe well
- Laugh
- Sing

Diabetes should be avoided whenever possible. If it has developed, then manage it as well as medical advice allows.

Keep weight within the recommended BMI range of 18 to 25. In particular, avoid obesity.

This section on the cardiovascular system has come to an end. We will now look at exercise, starting with the type aimed at the best for cardio-vascular health, which has the common name of "cardio" but is more accurately known as "aerobic."

CARDIO EXERCISE

Get on your bike, take up jogging, set up that gym membership—we are bombarded with such instructions. Why? What is the reason for all this encouragement, and if we are going to exercise, how should we do this?

As a fitness instructor, I need to be fit but also look the part. This is one of the reasons that I practice weight training to build muscle and stay fit and lean. If I showed up at a client's door 10 kg overweight and asked them to go on a diet, I doubt many people would believe I could help them live a healthy lifestyle!

So I have my own exercise routine, which is a combination of weight training (which I will discuss later) and cardio-vascular exercise for health, which we will look at now.

Cardiovascular exercise has, as its main goal, to keep us healthy by strengthening the cardio-vascular system. I am going to change the terminology here from "cardio" to "aerobic" as a better description of what is actually taking place. Aerobic exercise means "with air" and describes low- to moderate-intensity exercise that is usually performed over time and is dependent on an adequate supply of air to the body.

Solely aerobic exercise is on the low-intensity side, where all carbohydrates are aerobically turned into energy. This occurs via something called mitochondrial ATP production. Mitochondria use oxygen for the metabolism of carbohydrates, proteins, and fats. Exercises such as swimming, brisk walking, and jogging are all aerobic.

On the other hand, lifting heavy weights is not aerobic, as it requires such a high energy output that enough oxygen cannot be supplied to the muscle. The muscle just gets to the point of exhaustion, and then a rest period must take place.

In this case, muscles grow to accommodate this extra demand. It is as if the body says, "krikey, more demand is put on this muscle; the fibres have been stretched to their limit; I had better make it stronger."

Aerobic exercise works like this. Let us take the case of walking. A stroll through the woods on a summer's day will be beneficial, as we are getting fresh air into our system. If we then go from a stroll to a brisk walk, a number of things start to happen to our bodies. Most notable are an increase in the breathing rate and an increase in the heart rate. This is happening because the muscles in our legs, while we are on this "power walk," are saying, "Energy is getting low; send more fuel." And this fuel is supplied by the blood.

Remember, this is not weight training; we are not pushing the muscle to its limit. Rather, it is endurance, and as long as the body can supply energy via the blood supply, this leg muscle will continue to operate. Also, oxygen is required for metabolism, which is supplied by oxygenated blood reaching the muscles, which is why our breathing rate increases.

As the brisk walk continues and the pace is picked up, the heart rate and breathing rate continue to rise. A greater volume of blood is flowing through our vascular system. We can see from our discussion of cardiovascular disease that this helps prevent the formation of plaque on artery walls and thus keeps the arteries open.

The whole system is performing at a higher level than normal but is not overly stressed. As more energy is used in walking, waste heat is generated in our bodies, and so we start to feel warm and may sweat to control body temperature.

In cardio-aerobic exercise, our body is pushed a bit beyond its normal everyday energy output level, and our body adapts to this new demand. Again, it is as if the body says, "So we have to do this sort of thing now; I had better make the heart stronger; also, all this deep breathing is clearing out the lungs." A brisk walk for as little as 20 minutes, three times a week, provides measurable health benefits.

Some of the benefits of aerobic exercise are:

- The exercise causes an increase in the total number of red blood cells in the body, which are needed to move oxygen. This function alone reduces the incidence of anaemia and is particularly beneficial as people age.
- lowers the risk of heart disease, blood clots, and stroke.
- reduces blood pressure
- promotes weight loss by burning calories
- helps control blood sugar
- reduces diabetic risk
- strengthens bone
- lowers inflammation
- improves sleep
- strengthens the immune system

A healthy blood supply improves brain function by slowing the rate of neuronal loss caused by aging.

The above gives a good indication of the value of taking up aerobic exercise.

I will list some exercises that can be carried out and then explain why I recommend three in particular: walking, swimming, and cycling.

Aerobic exercises
- Jogging
- Team sports such as football, rugby, and basketball
- Gardening
- Cycling
- Walking briskly—enough to raise your heart rate and feel warm
- Swimming again at an intensity that raises the heart rate
- Dancing
- Skipping

All of the above will raise the heart and breathing rates, but in my opinion, some are better than others. I always think it is better to get into the habit of practising non-impact exercises. Swimming, for example, is a gentle, rhythmic exercise that has no impact on the joints. It is all smooth. Jogging, on the other hand, incurs an impact every time the foot hits the floor.

Why might this be a problem? The human body is a machine with bones, sinews, tendons, and muscles. At the intersection of one bone with another, such as the knee, a smooth cartilage acts to transfer forces from one bone to another. And this is all held in place by ligaments acting like straps or ropes. I like to think of the rigging used to hold the masts on ships in place. We want this joint mechanism to stay healthy.

Impacts may weaken the joint and, in some cases, lead to arthritis, bringing problems of pain and immobility. I know there is a discussion on the effect of impacts on joints, with many people believing there is no effect. It is clear that exercise is beneficial for overall health, and if the choice is to sit and do nothing or jog, I would say do some jogging. The reason for this is that the cardiovascular benefits outweigh possible damage to joints.

But a recent study backs up what I have just said about impacts [20]. Dr. Stehling pointed out that high-impact, weight-bearing activities are worse for knee health and carry a greater risk of injury over time. He went on to say, "Conversely, low-impact activities, such as swimming and cycling, may protect diseased cartilage and prevent healthy cartilage from developing disease."

This is why I believe it is better to stick to exercises that avoid strong impacts. Swimming is my favourite aerobic exercise, followed by cycling and a brisk walk. Rhythmic dancing is another good aerobic exercise.

You may recall that David initially refused to join a gym, preferring instead to control his weight through diet. I have advised him to do some aerobic exercise for his general health. He should ideally aim for three twenty-minute brisk walks per week. Also, a new sports facility with a heated swimming pool has opened in our town. I have advised him to at least try some swimming; we will see how it goes.

The key thing, I believe, for anyone trying to get fit and healthy is to give something a try and see if a good habit can be established.

MUSCULAR STRENGTH

At the time of writing, I am in my mid-twenties. As a young (ish) man, I want to look fit and healthy. This has a particular benefit for me as a fitness instructor, since I do need to look fit in order to inspire others in the same direction. In my everyday life, working with others, I do a lot of exercise, which enables me to stay fit in a cardiovascular fashion. Interestingly, it is possible to have very good cardiovascular fitness and yet not look particularly athletic. For the reasons mentioned above, I do need to look fit, so I have added muscular strength training to my own exercise routine. We will now discuss how to perform this strength training.

If you have ever watched films of the bodybuilder Arnold Schwarzenegger, you will notice that not only does he have large muscles, but they are also well defined and can be seen clearly under the skin. This definition is, to a large extent, caused by reduced body fat. However, the building of muscle itself is due to strength exercises coupled with a modified diet.

So, assuming the aerobic exercise is going well and the cardio-vascular fitness is taken care of, for those of you who wish to increase strength, read on. Otherwise, feel free to skip to the next section.

Working on the following three areas helps increase strength and muscle definition. These are

- Strength training exercises

- Diet

- Body fat reduction

We will take each of these in turn.

Strength training exercises

How do we grow a muscle and make it stronger? It's either use it or lose it. In fact, it is not just using the muscle, because everyday use will not make it grow. No, to grow a muscle, it must be pushed to its limit and exhausted.

Here is a story to illustrate. Milo of Croton, who appeared in the Olympic Games during the 6th century BC, was a superb wrestler and a six-time victor. He began weight training as a child by lifting a young calf. Then, on a daily basis, he carried on lifting the calf as it grew. By doing this, his muscles grew, and, again, it is said Milo was able to carry a fully grown ox on his shoulders into the Olympic stadium.

Now that would be quite a sight! Today we would name this technique "progressive overload training." Not only in weight training but in many areas of life, the following truth holds: small incremental changes over an extended period of time lead to unimaginable results.

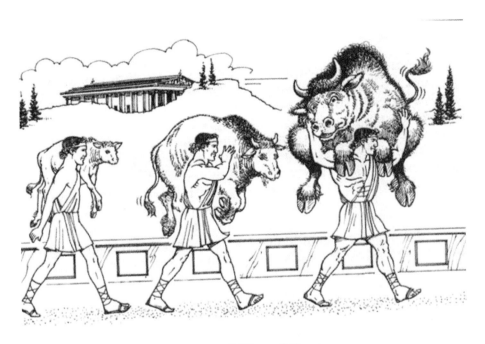

Figure. 5. Milo of Croton

So building muscle through weight training is nothing new. It is true that we know more today about how muscles work and the mechanical and chemical processes involved. But essentially, it is the same technique: push a muscle to exhaustion, and while it rests, it will grow. A good, high-protein diet is needed to grow this muscle; again, this was known in ancient times. I find it hard to believe, but it is said that Milo's daily diet consisted of 9 kg of meat, 9 kg of bread, and 10 litres of wine.

The muscles to grow in weight training are those that enable our body to move. The heart muscle is slightly different but will also grow with increasing demand placed upon it.

The process works for all joint moving muscles and illustrating one exercise will demonstrate the principle. This is how to grow the biceps muscle. This muscle is in the upper arm and enables us to bend our forearm upwards.

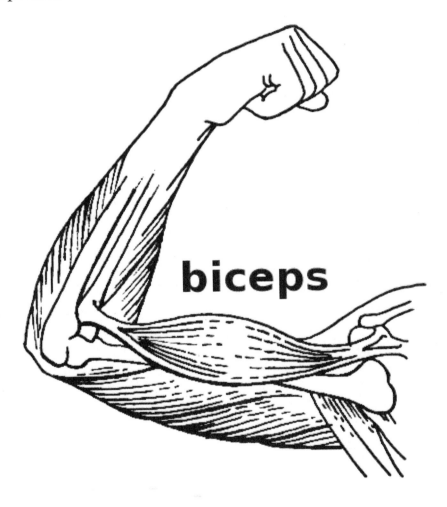

Figure. 6. Bicep Muscle

The bottom of the bicep is attached by a tendon to the radius bone in the forearm. The other end of the bicep is attached at the shoulder. When we decide to bend our elbow and lift our forearm, our brain sends a signal to the biceps muscle. This bicep muscle then contracts and pulls on the tendon attached at the radius, the elbow joint bends, and the forearm is raised.

If the weight we are lifting is light, such as a pen or cup of tea, then the muscle is not exhausted and can keep doing this many times—the muscle does not grow. However, if it is a heavy weight, then a number of striking things happen in the muscle. The muscle fibres are placed under high tension; this tells the body that the muscle needs to be stronger. Some muscle fibres can tear at high loads; again, this tells the body that the muscle needs to be stronger, which means bigger. Now for this bicep muscle to grow, it needs material—in the form of protein, and this protein comes from the diet, which I will come on to later.

It is worth considering that having larger muscles can provide us with health benefits other than just being stronger. In times of injury or illness, we need protein for repair, and in a crisis, our body can call on the material in our muscles to provide this. So having good muscle definition and lean body mass is good for our health.

A good maxim to have when building muscle is "train hard and eat plenty of protein."

Here is a biceps exercise. It is known as a bicep curl.

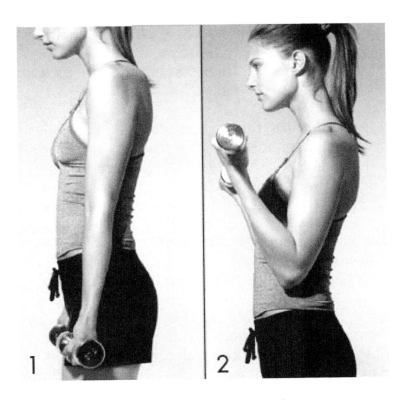

Figure. 7. Bicep Curl

- Select dumbbells of a weight that you can lift 10 times.
- Stand with your feet about an equal distance apart. Tensing your abdominal muscles
- Hold a dumbbell in each hand. Start with your arms relaxed at the sides of your body, with palms facing forward as shown in 1. Then go to 2, Bend at just the elbow joint and lift the weights so that the dumbbells touch your shoulders.

Your elbows should stay tucked in close to your ribs. Exhale while lifting.

- Lower the weights to the starting position in a gradual, controlled manner.
- Do this 10 times, then rest and do one or two more repetitions of 10 curls.

After this exercise, the biceps should feel well worked with a sense of exhaustion. A rest period is now required. Allow three days for this muscle to recover.

When we work at high intensity, we experience muscle damage. As mentioned, muscles grow when they are stressed and fed enough nutrients, meaning rest isn't the only component for muscle growth. We also need to make sure we are eating enough protein to build muscle mass.

Using my own training as an example, the exercise programme would go like this. If I worked the biceps on Monday, I will have to wait until Thursday before exercising them again. So on Tuesday and Wednesday, I can work on other muscles, such as the pectorals in the chest or the thigh muscles in the legs.

The biceps may feel painful during the rest period due to a build-up of lactic acid, which is produced in the muscle cells. It happens because the muscle has broken down carbohydrates for glucose during the bicep curls. Also, it takes some time for this lactic acid to be removed from the muscle, and this gives rise to soreness. Pain is also caused by the fact that the muscle has been stretched and the muscle fibres damaged. It can be seen as a signal from the body to leave this muscle alone for the time being.

A body building plan

Now, if I were to enter the gym and only work on one group of muscles such as forearms, then only those muscles would grow. I could end up looking a bit like Popeye, which would be a very strange look indeed!

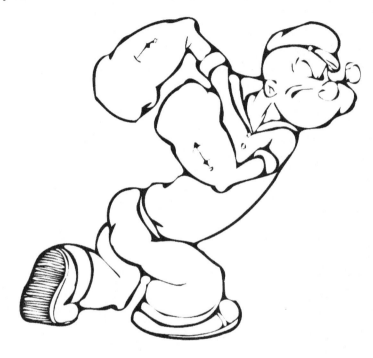

Figure. 8.

So we need a plan to work all the major muscle groups in the body.

I suggest exercising three times each week. Below is a suggested plan. To follow this programme effectively, a gym will be needed. Also, I very much advise that instruction be sought on how to do each exercise, the weight or tension to be used, and the number of repetitions.

It is very easy to overdo these exercises and cause unnecessary pain. However, having said that, a good effort needs to be put into these exercises to see results, but take instruction and take care.

To view any of these exercises on video - YouTube has many examples, a good one to have a look at is a list of exercises demonstrated with images of Arnold Schwarzenegger [21]. Also, a good text-based body workout plan can be found online at [22].

Monday: exercise programme 1
Tuesday: rest
Wednesday: exercise programme 2
Thursday: rest
Friday: exercise programme 3
Saturday: rest
Sunday: rest

The exercises in each programme are as follows:

Program 1
- Bench Press
- Lateral Pulldowns
- Squat
- Leg Curl
- Dumbbell Shoulder Press
- Bicep Curl
- Triceps Push

Programme 2

- Incline Dumbbell Press
- Rowing
- Leg Press
- Deadlift
- Lateral Raise
- Hammer Curl with Dumbbells
- Overhead Triceps Extension

Programme 3

- Cable Crossover
- Front lateral pulldown
- Leg Extension
- Seated Leg Curls
- Cable Pulls
- Preacher Curl

I realise this may seem like a great deal of work, so if a simpler start is needed, then I would recommend a weekend workout following Christiano Ronaldo [23]. In this YouTube video, Christiano goes through a good exercise routine that mainly follows the strength training philosophy, with the added benefit that there is no need for a gym.

As previously stated, eating protein and training hard is the way to go. So is there a need for dietary supplements, or can it be much simpler than that? Protein is essential for weight training. Eating the right foods and carefully timing meals ensures that you get the nutrients you need for a workout. This will maximise muscle growth after the workout is finished.

Not only protein but also carbohydrates and fat are necessary to provide energy, build muscle, and keep cells healthy.

For strength, consume 1.5 grams of protein per kilogramme of body weight per day. Add to this carbohydrates for energy, combined with plant-based fats where possible. But when to eat is important as well. Research suggests that proper timing can help muscle growth, coupled with recovery and tissue repair.

Also, it is important to consume enough calories each day, hence the need for carbohydrates, without which it is harder to build muscle. Keep in mind that strength training will mean that the body will need more energy than someone who is doing less exercise. So, keep an eye on the weekly weight and adjust accordingly.

Hydration is, as always, important, and there will be a need for this while training and also afterwards while the body recovers. As the body sweats, salt is lost. This must be replaced, and there are commercial drinks with just the right levels of electrolytes, carbohydrates, and proteins to accomplish this—but they are expensive.
In fact, there are three main types of sports drinks available, all of which contain various levels of fluid, electrolytes, and carbohydrates:

- isotonic
- hypertonic
- hypotonic

Isotonic drinks contain similar concentrations of salt and sugar as those in the human body. They quickly replenish fluids lost through sweating and provide a carbohydrate boost. This is the type of drink chosen by most athletes.

Hypertonic drinks contain a higher concentration of salt and sugar than the human body. These are drunk after exercise to boost carbohydrate intake and replenish muscle glycogen stores.

Hypotonic drinks contain a lower concentration of salt and sugar than the human body. They enable a quick input of fluid after sweating.

Most sports drinks tend to be isotonic. These contain around 2 teaspoons of sugar per 100 mL of drink.

If you wish to make up your own drink, then just follow this recipe. I always think it is great to be self-reliant, and it is good to know how to make our own energy drinks.

So what do we need? A good recipe needs to have the right level of carbohydrates; in this case, I will use sugar. Also, potassium needs to be replaced along with calcium and salt. This recipe uses a mix of coconut water and regular water to provide more flavour and to add some potassium (bananas are another good source).

The recipe adheres to nutritional guidelines, providing a 6% carbohydrate solution with 0.6 grammes of sodium per litre.

Grape and orange juice electrolyte drink
To make approximately 1 litre of

Ingredients:
0.25 tsp. salt
0.25 cup of grape juice
0.25 cup of orange juice
1.5 cups of coconut water
2 cups of cold water

Directions: Just put it all together and stir.

Many other recipes for these electrolyte-replacing drinks can be found online [24]. A variety of flavours will keep the motivation high, and knowing we are saving money along with having complete control over the ingredients helps greatly with that sense of self-reliance.

Body Fat

We have looked at the exercises needed for strength training and the diet, along with correct hydration. The third component is body fat control. There is a term in bodybuilding known as "cut," which refers to the look of a muscle when the body has a low percentage of fat. The reason the muscle can be seen clearly with clear indentations showing its structure is that the fat layer covering it is missing. Normally, we carry a layer of fat just below the surface of the skin, which obscures the visibility of the muscles. This is more pronounced in females, giving a softer look to the body.

Being "cut" is enabled by reducing body fat. We achieve this by limiting dietary fat. On a "cutting diet", we wish to reduce body fat but have enough protein to maintain muscle mass. To lose fat, we need to be on a calorie-deficient diet. When we do not have enough calories to maintain our body weight, our protein needs increase. This is true if we wish to maintain muscle mass. And remember, if we wish to look our best due to our dieting efforts, we need to lose fat while maintaining muscle mass—this is our goal.

To increase fat loss and avoid losing muscle mass, we increase the protein intake to 1.8 grams of protein per kilogramme of body weight. If we are on a very strict low-calorie diet or if we are already semi-ripped, we can increase our protein intake to 2.7 grams per kilogramme of body weight.

A word of caution This fat loss is a complex subject, and a good study needs to be done on the subject. We need to know what we are doing. Let us remember the title of this book is "Get Fit—Stay Fit." We want to get fit and stay that way as long as we can. We are going for longevity, not vanity. To do this, we are learning about the composition of the body and how it works. To be lean and muscular-looking may be an aim, but is it the healthiest? Let us digress and have a look at the function of fat in the body.

Having a store of fat helps in many ways. It is a store of energy that can be called upon if food becomes scarce. It provides insulation to keep us warm. Fat helps keep joints lubricated. Also, fat is a storehouse of hormones, particularly for women.

Obesity clearly causes the many problems mentioned earlier in this book. Obesity involves extra weight to carry, impact on joints, cardiovascular disease, and an increased risk of heart attacks and strokes. But having too little fat in the body—what is known as "essential fat"—also puts our health at risk. With a very low body fat level, the immune system is compromised, with studies showing an increase in heart disease and liver dysfunction. Also, too low a percentage of body fat in women can lead to infertility.

One extreme example of a bodybuilder who went too far with fat reduction is that of Andreas Munzer, who died in 1996. According to his autopsy report, he died of multiple organ failure and had almost no body fat [25]. He was known for having a very lean look, but it does appear that he went too far.

So let us stay in a healthy range. This range will depend to some extent on age and gender and, to a lesser extent, on our body shape.

For women, the lower end is 15 percent while young, rising to a healthy medium value of 24 percent at any age. When men are young, it is 8%, with a medium of 20% at any age. Below the lower levels, we may look leaner, but we need to be careful and take good advice. This Healthline link [26] has more information on the importance of fat levels in health.

Ok, well, it is good to know the acceptable fat levels, but how do we measure this? One of the simplest ways is to use an electronic weighing scale that can be programmed with height and weight to produce our BMI value.

Many of these bio-impedance scales also give water and fat percentages. It does this by having us stand barefoot on two metal pads and then measuring the resistance through our body. Because muscle, bone, and fat all have different resistance levels, the built-in algorithm can calculate the percentage of fat. Although some mistakes may occur as a result of excessive or insufficient hydration, the vast majority of us should be fine with these measurements.

However, there are other methods to measure body fat. As there is a layer of subcutaneous fat just below the skin, this can be measured with a pair of callipers, and then using a chart, the body fat percentage can be determined.

Ok, that will do for the strength training section. We have looked at how to build muscle, the adjustment to diet (mainly eating protein) needed to accomplish this, the need for hydration, and how to reduce and control body fat.

I hope by now the value of nutrition and exercise is clear for both cardiovascular fitness and strength training. The next section turns our attention to the dangers of just sitting around.

DANGER – WATCHING TV MIGHT KILL YOU

We may think that if we are exercising three times a week to the point of raising our heart rate and breathing rate, then we are doing pretty well in reducing the problems of sedentary living. After all, we are getting the heart and lungs working in order to enable and maintain that cardiovascular health that is so important to keeping fit.

However, if we then spend a lot of time sitting and hardly moving, there are potential problems that need highlighting. It is not so much that watching TV might kill you—but binge watching, say, a box set of Rome, Series 2, in which we hardly move for hours, could certainly be dangerous [27].

A 2016 study found that watching too much TV can increase the risk of venous thromboembolism, or the development of dangerous blood clots. A pulmonary embolism can be a deep vein thrombosis or a pulmonary embolism. Deep vein thrombosis often occurs in the deep veins of the legs. Pulmonary embolism, on the other hand, arises when a blood clot breaks away and moves to the lungs. This can be fatal.

So watching TV leads to reduced blood flow, particularly in the legs, which allows clots to form. This finding is not that surprising, for similar situations occur during any prolonged sitting. In particular, long-haul flights—longer than 4 hours—have also been linked with an increased risk of blood clot formation [28]. And as you would expect, the same clotting problem can occur on a long drive or train journey.

What can we do to prevent this dangerous situation? As mentioned, exercising three times a week is not enough. The problem is sitting without moving for hours. We have to get moving. The best thing to do is make sure to get out of the chair and walk around, even if it is just to get a glass of water. You may recall that while walking, the muscles in the legs are compressing the veins and moving blood back towards the heart. And staying hydrated in the right way is also important, for it has a preventive effect on blood thickening. Avoid alcoholic drinks, as these tend to have a dehydrating effect. This applies to both watching TV and flying.

If we find ourselves on a long car journey, then make planned stops at least once every hour. Break up motorway journeys and stop for twenty minutes; walk around.

A friend of mine does a lot of meditation in a seated position—he was once a monk! His morning routine, which used to be four hours, was broken up into an hour of meditation and then a half-hour break. During the break, he would ensure he had a drink and would walk around the garden, or his room if the weather was bad. He has never had any problems with circulation. So, sit like a monk!

I believe you get the picture—do not sit for more than an hour. We stay fit by understanding how our bodies work—learning about the machine we live in. Knowing about this machine known as the body allows us to maintain it and prevent problems from occurring.

BENEFITS OF WALKING AND SWIMMING

Having seen the benefits of moving the body to prevent clot formation, I now wish to consider two exercises of primary importance to health: walking and swimming. Swimming may not be for everyone, but assuming no disability, we can all take up walking. Here are the benefits:

Walking

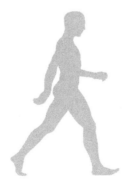

Figure. 9.

Getting up on our feet and walking helps us lose weight and become healthier. In particular, walking fast helps burn calories and improve heart health. Even a quick 10-minute walk every day improves health.

For the fast walks, before you start, wear comfortable shoes; trainers are fine but not essential. But even walking slowly around the house in slippers is OK. As mentioned, it is much better than sitting because the leg muscles are doing the work of moving the blood.

When out on a "proper" walk, aim to go faster than a stroll. The general rule is to walk at such a pace that you can still talk to a friend but would find singing more challenging. There are many walking apps for smartphones, which can give some motivating data. These indicate walking speed and distance. One of the most important things about any exercise is to make it a habit, and walking is no exception.

David is now incorporating a walk to the shops rather than taking his car. At first, it was novel and even felt inconvenient. But having done the shop walk a number of times, he reflected that he really enjoys the fresh air and the increased pulse and breathing rate. He said the walk made him feel alive. David tries to walk fast to raise his heart rate and breathing. He also tries to keep his body upright, swing his arms, and stretch out his legs to take longish strides. This all aids his overall fitness.

It is good practice to ask ourselves how we can increase walking, that important use of the legs.

"Is work within walking distance?"

"There is a lift, but why not use the stairs?"

"I am about to get in the car, but is my destination within walking distance?" Some people enjoy walking while listening to music or poetry. What would you like to hear?

Finally, walking is such a great general exercise that I wholeheartedly recommend it. It is such a preventative of ill health that we should all try to incorporate a good walk at least three times a week and, where possible, daily. Aim to just move around the house and not sit around for hours at a time. Let's get up on our feet!

Swimming

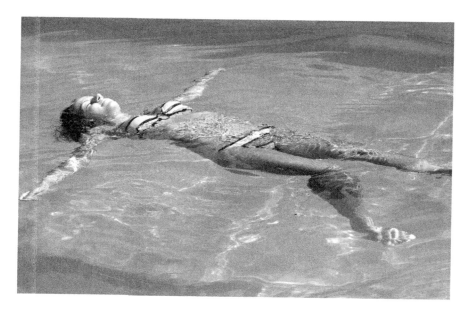

Figure. 10.

We are fortunate to have indoor, heated pools. Swimming is an activity that works our whole body. Do not worry about the style of swimming. Even doing a doggy paddle means we have to work our arms and legs. And as these are attached to our body, this helps to give us a whole-body workout as we activate our core muscles. If you are not very confident in the water, then most pools will provide instructors. Getting in the water is the important thing.

It is interesting that the body has to work quite hard against the water. This means that we are often exercising more intensely than we think—so we should take it easy at first. The buoyancy, along with the fact that we do not feel a sweating effect, can give the illusion that swimming is an easy option. So we can take our time and practice.

To finish this section, I just want to say that I recommend walking and swimming for everyone. However, if you have any concerns about your health, please consult your doctor.

CASE STUDY: JENNIFER

Jennifer is a professional woman in her fifties who approached me for assistance in losing weight. This is particularly important in that she suffers from type 2 diabetes, and her doctor has advised that she bring her weight into the normal BMI range.

Like many people, Jennifer has tried to lose weight in the past but failed, and this has left her feeling discouraged that further attempts will also fail. Clearly, one of my main tasks with Jennifer was motivating her to the point that she would succeed.

I mentioned to her the benefits of being at a normal weight. Normally, I list the disadvantages of being overweight first, but in Jennifer's case, I knew she needed an upbeat message right at the start. I told Jennifer that if she could bring her weight within the normal BMI range, then she could expect to receive the following five benefits:

These benefits are:

- Health benefits: in Jennifer's case with type 2 diabetes, better insulin response

- Feeling younger and more attractive

- Actually feeling better and having more energy

- Doing her bit for society—hopefully avoiding putting additional strain on others by managing her diabetes well and doing all she can to stay healthy.

- Life is less expensive—in Jennifer's case, eating less means lower food bills.

I did then go on to discuss the disadvantages of being overweight, just so we could acknowledge what she wished to avoid.

The disadvantages of being overweight are:

- Health problems—diabetes in Jennifer's case
- feeling unattractive (remember, we're trying to motivate not to make anyone feel bad). Jennifer said she had a lovely figure when she was young.
- feeling unhealthy and worrying over future health risks—sight and circulation problems associated with diabetes.
- Difficulties for society: we wish to avoid setting up problems for the future, that others may have to fix, and the burden may fall on our loved ones. Jennifer said she does not want to be a burden on her family and so wants to stay healthy for as long as she can.
- excessive cost, food itself, clothes, mobility.

We then went into fact-finding questions.

Age - 54 non smoker

high cholesterol and a BMI of slightly more than 27.

Exercise level: medium - Jennifer has a busy job as a nurse and is on her feet all day. She also keeps a well-maintained and clean house.

Diet: OK, but she needs to be careful with carbohydrates due to her diabetes. Jennifer does not drink alcohol.

Jennifer said she had the desire to lose some weight but was not sure how much.

We discussed her goals and came up with the following:

Reduce weight, aim for a BMI at the top end of the normal range, so 24 to 25, and in so doing improve cardio-vascular fitness.

I did a BMI calculation and found that for Jennifer's height, this would involve reducing her weight from 66 kg to 60 kg.

To achieve this, we used SMART goals.

- S-Specific: losing weight to a predetermined level in a predetermined amount of time, e.g., losing 6 kg.

- M-Measurable: aim for weight less than 60 kg

- A-Achievable, the weight loss is possible but not excessive.

- R-Relevant: it makes sense to lose this weight for diabetic health reasons. It is an appropriate weight loss for Jennifer.

- T-Time-Based: starting the programme in April 2022, we decided to achieve the goal by the New Year, a period of 8 months. So Jennifer will aim to get to 60 kg by this date, as the weight loss needed is less than 1 kg per month.

Following NHS guidelines, we came up with the following combination of diet and exercise:

Diet: Begin with a daily diet of 1300 calories, with more fibre from fruits and vegetables; follow the Eat Well guide. Drink zero-calorie cold drinks.

Exercise: Jennifer did not want to visit a gym or go swimming. As she works full time as a nurse and feels tired due to all the physical effort, Jennifer decided to not do any more exercise. Instead, she will manage the weight loss via diet alone.

Interview with Jennifer at the three-month interval

E is myself, Evander
J is Jennifer

E: Hello Jennifer
J: Hello Evander

E: So my first question is, How are you finding the diet? and what is the result after three months?

J: I have been a bit disappointed. If we look at my spreadsheet graph, we can see that I have lost less than 2 kg of weight, and this has taken me three months to achieve. I do not think I will reach my target weight by Christmas this year.

E: I am sorry to hear that you are disappointed. Can I put this into perspective for you? Firstly, you have lost weight, and it is very close to 2 kg. I notice from the chart that the weight is going up and down, but at no point have you gone above your starting weight. So your diet is having an effect, and you only have 4 kg more to lose to reach your target.

J: Thank you, Evander, I kept feeling like a failure, but your pointing out in particular that I have not gone above my starting weight is strangely uplifting. My biggest challenge is having to work long hours and eat when I can. This often means eating late in the evening when I come home from work. My husband usually has a meal ready for me.

E: How often do you weigh yourself?
J: Every Sunday, the moment I get up.

E: Would you be open to a couple of suggestions? Firstly, I would like you to weigh yourself every morning for the next two weeks. This will highlight if a spike upward occurs in the weight; if this happens, I would like you to consider why. Secondly, I would like you to record everything you eat and drink—a notebook is the best way to do this. Do you think you would be able to do this?

J: "Yes, Evander, I can do all of that." I really do want to lose this weight. It is for health reasons rather than vanity. As a nurse I know how the body functions. I want to use this knowledge to live long - longevity over vanity. I don't want to approach old age and realise I have added to my difficulties by not losing this weight.

E: That's great; I am pleased that you are on board with these suggestions. How are the family? Are they supportive of your weight loss endeavour?

J: They are all well. My husband is very supportive. In fact, he enters the data into the spreadsheet each Sunday. He also cooks my evening meal. I prepare my breakfast and lunch. My sons are in a world of their own. My youngest son, who is 22 years old, is home from university at the moment—it being the summer. I am worried about his weight—he is tall but heavy, with a BMI of over 35—definitely classed as obese.

E: It's encouraging to hear that your husband is pitching in. As for your youngest son, that BMI level is clearly a problem. I wonder if your attempt to lose weight will stimulate him to do the same.

J: Actually, that is a good idea. I realise that I do not talk about how I am trying to lose weight; I just keep it all to myself. I think I will talk with both my sons and tell them what I am trying to do and why. This may motivate the younger one to lose weight, and it might also motivate me to try a bit harder. If I can succeed, then he can as well.

E: Jennifer, that sounds like a fantastic idea. Do you think we need to adjust the diet, such as by setting the calorie intake a bit lower?

J: "No, I am happy with the way it is." My problem is that I have not stuck to the diet.

E: "Ok, it sounds like we are getting somewhere." I will give you a suggestion. The suggestion is to stick to breakfast, lunch, and dinner and not eat anything between those three meals. Also, make sure these three meals combined do not exceed the calorie limit of 1300 per day. If you stick to that, I guarantee that you will lose the weight and reach your target by Christmas.

J: Thank you, Evander; I do feel more positive now. When you arrived, I thought I had failed. Now, I see that it is all up to me; if I want to succeed, I can.

E: We have covered all you need, then. Shall we stop now?

J: "Yes, we can." We will be in touch mainly by text and email, but can I phone you if I need a motivation boost?

E: Yes, feel free to phone anytime; that is what I am here for.

J: "Ok, thank you once again."

GENDER IMPLICATIONS

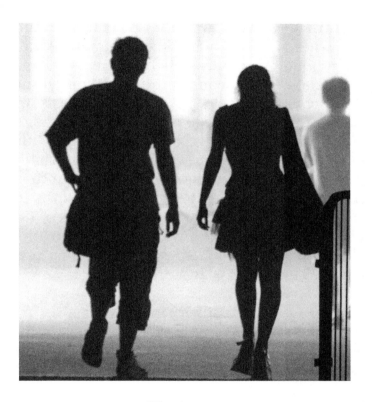

Figure. 11.

The two genders of male and female are most easily recognised by the way they look. Women tend to have a greater covering of subcutaneous fat, which adds to their feminine look. Men, on the other hand, can be rather angular, which is also a function of their body fat content.

Consequently, the minimum recommended fat levels are different for men (8 percent) and women (15 percent). This is only one difference, body fat level, but it will clearly affect the way a man or woman chooses to exercise and even the diet chosen.

There are many other considerations, and I will now just touch on one more.

The fact that women are the primary producers of children, where a pregnancy lasts nine months, at the end of which a bouncing 3 or 4 kg baby is created, has a major impact on their health considerations. Women must deal with the menstrual cycle on a monthly basis from the mid-teens to around the age of 50. The loss of blood with its stored iron at the end of each cycle puts a burden on the body. A lack of iron prevents the body from making enough red blood cells to carry oxygen around the system, and this needs to be done to replenish the loss. This can lead to iron deficiency anaemia, with feelings of tiredness, shortness of breath, and impaired concentration. This condition can also lead to a sense of being run down, accompanied by hair loss and brittle nails.

This tiredness is not surprising, as iron is primarily involved in energy production. Cells are helped by iron to turn energy from food into a source of energy the body can use. It helps keep the immune system healthy. Low levels of iron in the body result in a lower supply of oxygen to damaged cells, tissues, and organs. This weakens the ability to fight infection. Iron is also needed on the mental level. It enhances cognitive abilities including concentration, problem solving, and memory.

This mineral, the metal iron, which is so abundant in the world, cannot be produced by our bodies. Once it is lost, it must be replaced by food. The best source of iron is red meat, with lesser amounts found in chicken and fish. Iron is found in vegetables but is harder for the body to utilize. In particular, vegetarians and vegans need almost twice as much iron when considered on a daily quantity level. However, eating vitamin C-rich foods alongside iron-rich foods improves iron absorption.

Iron-rich vegetables are plentiful. Iron can be found in pulses, dark green vegetables, nuts, whole grains, and even dried fruits like figs and apricots.

All of this discussion tells us why women need more iron in their diets, for it ensures the loss bound up in the blood cells is replaced.

But menstruation does come to an end at menopause, usually somewhere in the fifth decade. At this stage of life, the iron requirement for men and women even out. If you are a woman, where you are in the cycle of life is an important consideration, and as always, my advice for a female wishing to go on a fitness programme is to consult their doctor.

Moving on to a consideration of men. is there anything in their genetics that they need to watch out for? I will point to two conditions here: heart disease and type 2 diabetes.

First, heart disease: it is not all prevented by good exercise and diet. Mental health comes into play here. Men have traditionally kept their stress bottled up. Society conditions them that way. I heard a little boy recently, who was a bit tearful, being told to "man up" by his older brother. Such instruction may aid in the development of an individual who appears to the outside world to be a man in command, but on the inside, it's a different story. Outside, he appears to be a big, strong man, but on the inside, he is a scared little boy who never grew past the age of six. The conflicts between inner and outer life create tension in the body.

Put simply, stress is a killer. This consideration is backed up by a recent scientific study [29]. Thousands of participants between the ages of 18 and 30 were followed for more than 30 years. The analysis found more than 20% of participants experienced a high rate of exposure to damaging childhood events, and those participants had health issues throughout their adult lives. "The results of this study further confirm that cardiovascular disease is not simply a problem at older ages but has its origins in childhood experiences," said Karestan C. Koenen, a professor at Harvard University.

The data is clear: more men die of heart disease than any other cause of death. So, as well as eating a balanced diet, including fruits and vegetables, quitting smoking, and doing enough exercise, stress needs to be managed. It may be the case that medication to handle the mood is needed. A man needs to have regular checkups without being all "manly" and putting them off. Also, use doctor visits to check blood pressure and have blood tests to monitor cholesterol. The aim is to detect heart problems before they become serious.

Moving on to type 2 diabetes in men. Men have a higher risk of getting type 2 diabetes than women, even at a lower weight. This is partly due to male bodies having more belly fat, which is identified as a major risk with this disease. Considering that men generally have lower body fat than women, the excessive belly fat is even more disproportionate. A beer belly needs to be eliminated by managing weight and getting more exercise. Just doing this will reduce the risk. My advice is to see a doctor and have a pre-diabetic check.

This has been a very cursory look at gender implications; there are many issues not touched on here. All I would like you to take away from this is that men and women are different in their bodies and minds, and this needs to be reflected in how they approach health and fitness.

HEALTH IN ADVANCING YEARS

To grow old with a fit and healthy body, free from strain or pain, is a future I wish for myself—and, for that matter, all humanity. However, for many of us, this is not a guarantee, as there are many diseases and ailments that can appear apparently out of nowhere. A friend of mine once sang a song: "A for angina, B for bronchitis, C for cancer, D for diabetes, and so on." There is much illness and pain in the world, causing all kinds of suffering. We cannot escape it all; it is part of the human condition.

Be that as it may, there are clearly things we can do to gain a greater chance of healthy aging. For one thing, following the guidelines in this book—healthy eating, weight control, cardio-vascular fitness, avoiding excessive alcohol consumption, and not smoking—sets us up well for illness prevention. Controlling one metric, body weight, is extremely beneficial to health, particularly diabetes.

According to science [30], "Research shows strong links between a high BMI and type 2 diabetes, with the risk of the condition rising with increasing BMI." A review of over 12,000 people in the United States published in 2014 showed that people with a BMI of 25–29.9 had a 50% increased risk of diabetes compared to people with a BMI of 18.5-24.9. Obesity was linked with increased rates of diabetes between 2.5 and 5 times higher than people of normal weight, with the highest risk being those with a BMI of 40 or more.

Further, the World Health Organization states that a high BMI is a major risk factor for heart disease, stroke, bone and joint problems, including osteoarthritis, and a number of cancers, including breast, colon, and endometrial cancer.

Perhaps it is best not to list all the problems of smoking and excessive alcohol consumption, as I do not wish to frighten anyone. So let me round this bit out by just saying that the person who is heavily overweight, drinks plenty, smokes, does not exercise and eats poorly is putting their chances of living to a healthy old age in danger.

There are no guarantees, but, on the other hand, someone who controls their weight, has a healthy diet, takes exercise, does not smoke, and controls alcohol consumption has a much higher chance of staying healthy and reaching old age. Moreover, they are healthy, without pain, enjoy their retirement years, and live longer.

Here are a few conditions to watch out for: I will just list physical problems and go on to mental stuff in the next chapter.

- Arthritis
- Cancer
- Diabetes
- Heart disease
- Osteoporosis
- Respiratory diseases

Let us look at each of these in turn, their descriptions, and what helps prevent them.

Arthritis:
Description: Osteoarthritis is the most common type of arthritis and tends to affect people in their mid-40s or older. It is more prevalent in women. The condition affects the smooth cartilage lining of joints, making movement more difficult than usual. It causes discomfort and stiffness. Once the cartilage lining starts to roughen and thin out, this can cause swelling and the formation of bony spurs called osteophytes. In extreme cases, the cartilage is lost and the bones contact each other. This increases pain and can lead to bone loss and deformation of the joint.

Prevention: Avoid obesity, as this increases the strain on weight-bearing joints such as the knees, hips, and spine. Also, wear comfortable shoes that have a soft, springy sole and heel. Although exercise is important, excessive weight bearing on joints or impacts should be avoided. So as we age, we may need to lay off the weights and the running. As mentioned before, two great exercises are walking and swimming.

Cancer:
Description: As we go through life, each of the millions of cells in the body needs replacing. Cancer occurs when cells grow and reproduce incorrectly. These out-of-control cells can then invade parts of the body and grow uncontrollably, resulting in tumours and impairing the function of organs. According to the NHS [31], there are more than 200 cancers, the most common of which are breast, lung, prostate, and colon.

Prevention: There is much research ongoing to find the causes of cancer and hence its prevention. Lifestyle does play a factor, and certain things are best avoided. We know of the dangers of tar and chemicals in smoking that are linked to lung cancer. However, the fact that chemical exposure can cause cancer has been known for hundreds of years.

Cancer among chimney sweeps emerged in England, a cold country traditionally heated by coal fires. In 1775, Percival Pott identified scrotal cancer in men as being due to their occupation. At this time, climbing boys were used for the narrow English chimneys. Up they would go, sometimes naked, and get covered in soot. Hygiene was uncommon—perhaps a bath once a year. Stephen found that this was the first reported form of occupational cancer [32].

Percival commented, "The fate of these people seems peculiarly hard... They are treated with great brutality... They are thrust up narrow and sometimes hot chimneys, where they are bruised, burned, and almost suffocated, and when they get to puberty, they become "liable to a most noisome, painful, and fatal disease." In 1788, laws were changed to require boys to be at least 8 years old and to wear protective clothing.

By 1840, the recommendations were even more beneficial to health, stating that those under 21 not be employed in the trade. Consequently, there was a reduction in this type of cancer.

This history showed us that there are things we can do with our lifestyle to help avoid developing cancer. I accept that not many of us are climbing up the insides of dirty chimneys and getting covered in coal dust. But people do smoke; they put the tar and chemicals into their lungs, and they pay money to do it! So number one is to avoid smoking. Also, getting too much ultraviolet light can cause skin cancer, so we wear hats and cover our skin with factor 7. Eating too much red meat is linked to colon cancer, so moderation here would make sense. Above all, exercise, eating a good diet, and weight control are some of the best hedges against developing cancer.

Diabetes
Description: As I am talking about life in advancing years,
I will examine type 2 diabetes, which also covers 90
percent of all diabetic cases. Type 2 diabetes is where the
pancreas either does not manufacture enough insulin or
the insulin it produces does not work properly. Insulin is
needed to enable blood glucose to enter cells and fuel our
body.

The condition leads to high blood sugar, which has a
damaging effect on the heart and small blood vessels such
as those found in the kidneys, eyes, and feet. The
situation is such that there can be high levels of sugar in
the blood from all the digested food, yet the fact that it
cannot get into the cells to fuel them results in tiredness.
It's similar to having a full tank of gas but being unable to
start the engine.

The risk factors for developing type 2 diabetes are
increasing age, weight (particularly around the middle),
and diet. Also, ethnicity plays a part. Afro-Caribbeans and
black Africans are more vulnerable than white Europeans.

Prevention: We have no control over our ethnicity or age
because they were set in motion at birth. However, there
is much we can do to prevent the onset of type 2 diabetes
and, even if it has developed, put it into remission. It will
come as no surprise to the readers of this book that diet,
weight control, and exercise are the way to go.

Weight control means getting into a BMI range below 25.
Exercise—do that brisk walking to get the pulse rate up
and a little out of breath. Diet is a more specific term. It is
important to eat a balanced diet with reduced
carbohydrates, as this has a tendency to quickly raise
blood sugar.

Higher-fiber carbohydrates are more beneficial as they are slower to digest. Whole-grain bread, brown rice, and whole-wheat pasta are all good options within a diabetic diet. Calorie control is equally important for preventing body weight gain. I recommend weighing once a week; Sunday morning before breakfast works for me.

Heart Disease
Description: You may recall there is a whole section on this in the chapter, "Cardio Vascular Fitness." So I will just give a quick recap here. The heart is a pump—quite mechanical in its operation—pushing the blood around the body. The blood is like a transport system, moving all the nutrients into the cells and enabling waste material to be removed. If this pump goes wrong, we are in trouble. Coronary artery disease (CAD) is one of the most common causes of death in the UK. The risk increases as we grow older and gain weight. CVD is avoided in many cases by making healthy lifestyle choices. Again, diet, weight control, and exercise can be extremely beneficial in later life.

Osteoporosis
Description: More common in women than men, osteoporosis is effectively a weakening of the skeletal system. After menopause in women and andropause in men, the hormonal changes result in a lessening of bone mass in the body. As a result of this loss, bones become more fragile, making them prone to fracture. Often, the older person does not know they have osteoporosis until they fall and break a bone—the hip, forearm bone, or spinal vertebrae.

Prevention: As the condition presents itself with a broken bone, which happens typically after a fall, avoiding falls is paramount. As we age, we can install more handrails around our home, fix loose carpets, and wear good, comfortable, and stable shoes, all with the aim of reducing the chance of a fall. Exercise and keeping weight down are always helpful, as is a good diet with increased protein. Exercise in particular will keep the muscles in good shape, which is necessary for good balance and control of movement. Avoid smoking and limit alcohol consumption. Vitamin D and calcium supplements in the diet can help maintain bone density.

Respiratory Diseases
Description: This is all to do with the lungs, those organs responsible for getting oxygen into our system and carbon dioxide out. Chronic obstructive pulmonary disease (COPD), including emphysema and bronchitis, all result in a weakening of this gaseous exchange. Lung cancer compromises the function of the respiratory system, and the cancer can spread to other parts of the body. All these conditions weaken the body, leading to disability and death.

Prevention: In each case, the risk of developing any of these conditions is increased by smoking. In the case of lung cancer, 70 percent of people who develop the disease are smokers. The number one prevention, then, is to not smoke. Getting the breathing rate up via exercise expands and eliminates stale air from the bottom of our lungs. Hydration is also very important; on a cold day, when we breathe out, this moist air can be seen to immediately condense into a mist. So we are losing fluid all the time through our lungs, and we need to drink to maintain hydration.

From all this, it is clear that as we age, there is a greater risk of developing any of the above conditions. But there are things we can do to help ourselves. With the danger of sounding like an old record, we are more likely to stay healthy if we keep our body weight within the normal BMI range of 18 to 25. To do this, we need to watch our diet and eat healthy—neither too much nor too little. Build in a good exercise plan, even if it is just brisk walking a few times each week. Do not smoke! Control alcohol. A few bottles of beer a week or a glass of wine now and again may be beneficial, but too much and we are increasing the risk of disease.

Okay, the repetition of this message of weight loss, diet, exercise, no smoking, and alcohol control may be getting annoying. It is going to take a bit of work to develop as a habit. Where are habits formed? in the brain—so let's take a look at this amazing organ that we all have but have never seen.

BRAIN HEALTH

What I am going to look at here is the physical organ called the brain and what we can do to keep it healthy. The mind, which we are, consciousness, awareness, and motivation, I will be treating as something different but definitely linked to brain functioning.

All I will cover for the mind is motivation, a needed quality on our road to getting fit and staying that way.

So first, the physical brain. It weighs about 3 lbs. and sits within our skull. It has no muscles and instead is made up of neurons, has a blood supply, and is bathed in fluid. It has the consistency of stiff, jelly-like custard. In fact, the brain can be thought of as being made up of three brains, the hindbrain, midbrain, and forebrain, as shown overleaf.

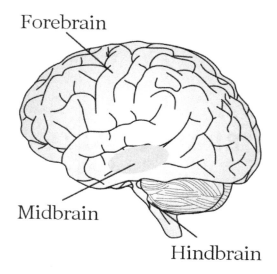

Figure. 12. The Human Brain

Each of these brains can be thought of as a branch on an evolutionary tree. The hindbrain controls basic functions such as breathing and heart rate while also being responsible for fine motor movement. We share this hindbrain with many animals. It is the midbrain and the forebrain that develop further in what can be considered higher animals, such as the chimpanzee and humans.

The midbrain sits on top of the hindbrain and, although small in size, is complex, being responsible for multiple life functions. It controls some reflex actions, such as involuntary eye movements or other motor movements. When we hear a loud sound and jump, it is the midbrain that has initiated this. The same applies to touching a very hot or cold surface and reflexively pulling the hand away. The midbrain is also responsible for heat regulation, the sleep cycle, and dopamine regulation. We will look at dopamine in more detail later, as it is important for motivation.

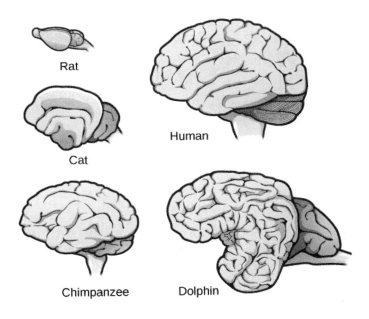

Rat

Cat

Human

Chimpanzee   Dolphin

Figure. 13. Other Brains

The forebrain contains the cerebrum, a convoluted structure with many folds. These folds give the brain a greater surface area than would normally be the case for a smooth ball inside a case—the skull. In fact, many other animals do not have these folds—or at least not to this extent. It is in the forebrain that the complexity of language, thought, and imagination take place. Some would even say it is where we, as individuals, reside. The forebrain is divided into right and left hemispheres. The right is associated with imagination, while the left tends to be language and logical thought—the seat of reason.

Admittedly, these are crude divisions—there is, of course, far more complexity to the left and right sides of the brain, but enough for us to consider here.

Each hemisphere controls the other side of the body. If we have ever met someone who has had a stroke, we will notice this immediately. If they have right-side weakness coupled with difficulty forming or understanding words, we can accurately predict that the stroke has occurred in the left hemisphere of the brain.

For more information on brain structure and function, a good reference can be found online [33].

With the brain being such an important organ, we would like to keep it as healthy as we can for as long as we can. There is no reason why, with a bit of care, we cannot live with an actively healthy brain, allowing us the ability to keep learning and enjoying life right into old age.

So how do we keep this brain healthy? Stroke and dementia are the two physical illnesses that most people wish to avoid. We will look at each in turn.

Stroke:
To quote from the NHS website [34], "A stroke is a serious, life-threatening medical condition that happens when the blood supply to part of the brain is cut off." When this happens, neurons in the affected area cease to function due to the lack of oxygen and glucose and begin to die quickly, within a few minutes. This is the reason why, if we observe someone having a stroke, we need to act fast and get emergency aid. You may have seen advertisements for stroke treatment that use the acronym

FAST.
- F: Face. Is the mouth or eye looking droopy?
- A: Arms: the person cannot move one of their arms.
- S: Speech is slurred.
- T: Time is of the essence; get help.

There are two main types of stroke. An ischaemic stroke occurs when a blood vessel leading to a part of the brain becomes blocked; approximately 85% of all cases are caused by this. This is why, when alerted to a patient having a stroke, the medical emergency team will often give clot-busting medicine to dissolve the clot and get the blood moving again. In 85% of cases, they will have made the right decision. I should also mention transient ischemic attacks (TIAs), in which the blood temporarily stops flowing. These do not cause permanent damage to neurons but are an indication that the blood transport system is impaired.

The other type is when a blood vessel breaks open and can no longer deliver the blood to the neurons; instead, the blood leaks into the surrounding tissue. The neurons that are now starved of oxygen and glucose stop functioning and begin to die. A further complication is that the blood that is leaking into the surrounding tissue is poisonous. It will damage the neurons there, further adding to the difficulties the brain is experiencing.

What makes someone more prone to a stroke?

There are a number of factors.

- Increasing age
- High blood pressure
- High cholesterol
- Heartbeat irregularity
- Diabetes
- Smoking
- Drinking too much alcohol
- Obesity

The health advice is the same as it has been many times before. Control weight with exercise and a healthy diet; don't smoke; and drink alcohol in moderation.

One aspect of cholesterol control may necessitate the use of a medication such as a statin. This will depend on the individual, as some people may have a genetic disposition to create more cholesterol than others.

Dementia:
Alzheimer's can be considered synonymous with dementia, while it is in fact just one type. The definition of dementia given by Dementia Uk [35] is that "dementia is an umbrella term for a range of progressive conditions that affect the brain." Now that sounds like a very broad term, and so it is. There are many physical conditions that affect brain health and the way we therefore function, and these can become progressively more problematic.

The five most common types of dementia in order from high to low are:

- Alzheimer's
- Vascular
- Lewy body
- Frontotemporal
- Mixed (for example, Alzheimer's and vascular)

As mentioned, dementia is an umbrella term, and there are more than 200 subtypes of dementia. The cause of many of these is still unknown. The prevalence of dementia increases with age, and there can be genetic involvement in some cases. There are no guarantees that a particular individual will not suffer from dementia, and the risk increases with age. However, vascular dementia is something we can do something about. It often follows a stroke or history of TIAs, and therefore, living a healthy lifestyle as outlined in this book is a very good policy to take.

The mind:
When we think of the mind, we do not necessarily think of the physical brain, but rather more the flavour of our experience. Happiness, joy, sadness, depression, a racing mind full of thoughts, or not knowing what to say at a party are all experiences we know.

For our purposes here, I just want to talk about motivation and how to achieve it. Dopamine is a neurotransmitter. Dopamine tells us how well things are going regarding obtaining a reward. This helps us decide how hard to work toward a goal. When dopamine is high, we are not put off by setbacks; instead, we learn from our mistakes. So how can we increase the dopamine in our brains? We do this by living the healthy lifestyle described here. But additionally, we need to ensure we get enough sleep and do things we enjoy. There is evidence that spending time in the open air increases dopamine.

Motivation is also enhanced by keeping the goal in mind. Take the case of David—his goal was defined as "reach the target weight of 11 stone by his 66th birthday." He is using smart goals to achieve this. Specific, measurable, achievable, realistic, and time-based. He weighs himself once a week and keeps a spreadsheet of the results. He watches motivational YouTube videos of people who have succeeded in losing weight. He also takes note of the warnings about smoking and excessive drinking. All this is motivational and has a direct effect on his mind—it raises the dopamine level. The physical brain is being kept healthy by mental activity. So do things that make you happy; it is good for you.

TO CONCLUDE

I wish you all the very best in achieving your health and fitness goals. If you follow the simple guidelines in this book, look for inspiration via motivational books and videos, stay focused, and keep the goal in mind, success is assured.

I will repeat it one more time. To have a long healthy life - longevity over vanity we need to learn about the body and do the following.

- Diet - Mediterranean is good
- BMI - get into the normal range
- Exercise - get the heart rate and breathing up
- Do not smoke
- Moderate alcohol consumption

If you would like help setting goals for weight, fitness, and health, feel free to contact me. I can be contacted to set up a session to determine the goal and timeframe, as well as a guideline for what needs to be adjusted in the client's lifestyle. I also provide ongoing guidance.

with very best wishes
Evander Sampson

REFERENCES

[1] https://www.nhs.uk/mental-health/conditions/anorexia/overview/ accessed 10 June 2022

[2] https://www.nhs.uk/conditions/hypother2omia/ accessed 10 June 2022

[3] https://www.medicalnewstoday.com/articles/body-fat-percentage-chart#problems-and-limitations accessed 10 June 2022

[4] https://www.nhs.uk/live-well/healthy-weight/bmi-calculator/ accessed 16 June 2022

[5] https://www.nhs.uk/conditions/obesity/ accessed 16 June 2022

[6] https://www.independent.co.uk/arts-entertainment/films/news/marlon-brando-superman-cary-elwes-b1973521.html accessed 16 June 2022

[7] https://www.nhs.uk/Livewell/Goodfood/Documents/The-eatwell-Guide-2016.pdf Accessed 16 June 2022

[8] https://www.calculator.net/bmr-calculator.html accessed 16 June 2022

[9] https://www.nhs.uk/live-well/healthy-weight/bmi-calculator/ accessed 16 June 2022

[10] https://www.nhs.uk/live-well/eat-well/why-5-a-day/ accessed 16 June 2022

[11] https://www.healthline.com/nutrition/2000-calorie-diet accessed 16 June 2022

[12] https://www.nhs.uk/conditions/vitamins-and-minerals/ Accessed 20 October 2022

[13] https://www.youtube.com/watch?v=G06HY051-NQ Accessed 20 October 2022

[14] https://www.sleepfoundation.org/how-sleep-works/benefits-of-sleep Accessed 20 October 2022

[15] https://www.nhs.uk/live-well/sleep-and-tiredness/ Accessed 20 October 2022

[16] https://www.mayoclinic.org/healthy-lifestyle/adult-health/expert-answers/heart-disease-prevention/faq-20057986 Accessed 25 August 2022

[17] https://www.amazon.co.uk/How-We-Die-Sherwin-Nuland/dp/009947641X Accessed 4 August 2022

[18] https://www.nhs.uk/conditions/coronary-heart-disease/causes/ Accessed 11 August 2022

[19] https://www.nhs.uk/live-well/exercise/exercise-guidelines/physical-activity-guidelines-for-adults-aged-19-to-64/ Accessed 11 August 2022

[20] https://www.webmd.com/osteoarthritis/news/20091130/too-much-exercise-may-pose-arthritis-risk Accessed 25 August 2022

[21] https://www.youtube.com/watch?v=pCFVZexvQKY Accessed 6 October 2022

[22] https://muscleevo.net/full-body-workout/ Accessed 6 October 2022

[23] https://www.youtube.com/watch?v=QvbpeETBoGg Accessed 6 October 2022

[24] https://www.healthline.com/health/fitness-exercise/homemade-electrolyte-drink#recipe Accessed 13 October 2022

[25] https://en.wikipedia.org/wiki/Andreas_M%C3%BCnzer Accessed 13 October 2022

[26] https://www.healthline.com/health/exercise-fitness/ideal-body-fat-percentage Accessed 13 October 2022

[27] https://www.medicalnewstoday.com/articles/321002 Accessed 20 October 2022

[28] https://www.healthline.com/health/blood-clots-and-flying#symptoms Accessed 20 October 2022

140

[29]
https://www.heart.org/en/news/2020/04/28/traumatic-childhood-increases-lifelong-risk-for-heart-disease-early-death
Accessed 10 November 2022

[30] https://www.diabetes.co.uk/bmi/why-is-bmi-important.html Accessed 24 November 2022

[31] https://www.nhs.uk/conditions/cancer/
Accessed 24 November 2022

[32]
https://en.wikipedia.org/wiki/Chimney_sweeps%27_carcinoma
Accessed 24 November 2022

[33] https://www.ninds.nih.gov/health-information/public-education/brain-basics/brain-basics-know-your-brain
Accessed 15 December 2022

[34]
https://www.nhs.uk/conditions/stroke/
Accessed 15 December 2022

[35] https://www.dementiauk.org/about-dementia/dementia-information/what-is-dementia/
Accessed 15 December 2022

Helpful books that can be found on Amazon UK

Motivation-Bounce: The Myth of Talent and the Power of Practice

The Fitness Mindset: Eat for energy, Train for tension, Manage your mindset, Reap the results

Also there is this online resource:
The Eatwell Guide: helping you eat a healthy, balanced diet. This is a free NHS PDF, easily findable via Google. The full link to this online information is https://www.nhs.uk/livewell/goodfood/documents/the-eatwell-guide-2016.pdf.

List of figures

https://free-
images.com/display/dumbbell_bicep_curls.html
desaturated

Figure. 8. Popeye
https://free-
images.com/display/popeye_spinach_sailor_man.html

Figure. 9. Walking
https://commons.wikimedia.org/wiki/File:Silhouette_of
_a_walking_man.svg Mette Aumala, CC0, via Wikimedia
Commons (de-saturated)

Figure. 10. Swimming
https://commons.wikimedia.org/wiki/File:Woman_enjo
ys_a_swimming_pool.JPG Tibor Végh, CC BY 3.0
(de-saturated)

Figure. 11. Man and Woman
https://commons.wikimedia.org/w/index.php?search=m
an+and+woman&title=Special:MediaSearch&go=Go&typ
e=image Fred Bchx from Tournai, Belgique, CC BY 2.0
<https://creativecommons.org/licenses/by/2.0>,   via
Wikimedia Commons (Cropped)

Figure 12 The Brain
https://commons.wikimedia.org/wiki/File:Human-
brain-vector.svg Unknown author (de-saturated)

Figure. 13. Other Brains
https://commons.wikimedia.org/wiki/File:Figure_35_0
3_05.jpg   CNX   OpenStax,   CC   BY   4.0
<https://creativecommons.org/licenses/by/4.0>,   via
Wikimedia Commons (cropped and de-saturated by
Stephen Small)

ABOUT THE AUTHORS

Evander Sampson is a personal fitness instructor offering guidance in nutrition and exercise. He works in the West of England. Evander experienced health issues while young - involving a weak lung development. Prompted by this he has worked steadily on his own health and is now fit, healthy and strong. He wishes to show others the way to health.

Qualifications
HNC Sports Science
Personal Training Diploma in Lifetime Training

Contact
      email: evander16and@live.com
      mobile: 07795538734
      home: 01225 971690

Stephen Small is a lifetime learner. His most recent qualification is a BSC in Psychology which Evander made good use of while the chapter on the Brain and Motivation were being compiled. Stephen typed up, proof read and typeset the manuscript. He also sourced all the images from the public domain, giving credit to authors where possible. If he has missed any attribution he will gladly correct this. All images were de-saturated and some were cropped.

Printed in Great Britain
by Amazon

21243733R00088